SUCCESS AND THE SPIRIT

AN AQUARIAN PATH TO ABUNDANCE

Lectures and Meditations by Yogi Bhajan
Siri Singh Sahib of Sikh Dharma and Master of Kundalini Yoga

Kundalini Research Institute
Training ∞ Publishing ∞ Research ∞ Resources

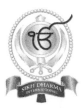

© 2011 Sikh Dharma International
www.sikhdharma.org

Published by the Kundalini Research Institute
Training → Publishing → Research → Resources
PO Box 1819
Santa Cruz, NM 87567

www.kundaliniresearchinstitute.org

ISBN 978-1-934532-74-4

The diet, exercise and lifestyle suggestions in this book come from ancient yogic traditions. Nothing in this book should be construed as medical advice. Any recipes mentioned herein may contain potent herbs, botanicals and naturally occurring ingredients which have traditionally been used to support the structure and function of the human body. Always check with your personal physician or licensed health care practitioner before making any significant modification in your diet or lifestyle, to insure that the ingredients or lifestyle changes are appropriate for your personal health condition and consistent with any medication you may be taking. For more information about Kundalini Yoga as taught by Yogi Bhajan please see www.yogibhajan.org and www.kundaliniresearchinstitute.org.

This publication has received the KRI Seal of Approval. This Seal is only given to products that have been reviewed for accuracy and integrity of the sections containing 3HO lifestyle teachings and Kundalini Yoga as taught by Yogi Bhajan*.

Editor: SS Ek Ong Kaar Kaur Khalsa
Production Editor: Sat Purkh Kaur Khalsa
Copy Editor: Gurbani Kaur
Cover Design and Layout: Prana Projects: Ditta Khalsa, Biljana Spasovska
Photography: Ravitej Singh Khalsa, Khalsa Marketing Group
Model: Guru Nam Kaur
Back Cover Photo Credit: Gurumustuk Singh Khalsa

Dedication

This book is dedicated to all those who never met Yogi Bhajan in his lifetime, but who have a destiny to understand, practice and share his teachings.

May you find a genuine connection with your spirit. May you walk the path of your destiny. May you rise to the challenge of time and space. And may peace, prosperity and happiness blossom wherever you go.

Aquarian Age Prosperity Affirmation

Prosperity, prosperity, prosperity is perpetual with people who prefer to be penetrating, prepared and purposeful. But prosperity only comes to those who are trustworthy, those who deliver and those who are content and consistent. Basically, it boils down to commitment. If you put your soul into anything, you can win the whole world. It will be yours. You can sweep prosperity with your commitment. Contain, commit and be continuous.

∾ *Siri Singh Sahib Bhai Sahib Harbhajan Singh Khalsa Yogiji*

TABLE OF CONTENTS

KRIYAS, MEDITATIONS & SHABADS

SELF-CREATED PEOPLE

Five hundred years ago, in what is now Northern India and Pakistan, a very quiet revolution of the spirit began. A teacher by the name of Guru Nanak[1] started sharing some incredibly radical ideas: that women should be educated and treated with honor and respect; that every religion comes from the same Creator—therefore the highest religion is to acknowledge our common brotherhood and sisterhood; that people have the right to earn their own living and enjoy the benefits of their own labor; that caste and class should not be an obstacle to a person's livelihood or self-expression; and that developing a meditative mind—capable of seeing the light of the Divine in all people—could unlock the full potential of the human being.

Radical as his ideas were at the time, Guru Nanak's teachings attracted a community of people dedicated to doing things differently. Over the course of the next 250 years, nine other teachers succeeded Guru Nanak, and continued to build on his foundation. The result was a revolution from within. Towns and communities formed where people from different religions lived in harmony and worked together, side by side. Women received educations and were sent out to teach others. People worked together, regardless of what caste they were born into. What they earned, they shared with one another. Meditating together every morning and evening, they touched the God within and manifested their inner potential.

Inevitably, these communities became incredibly prosperous and successful. They didn't conquer and exploit territories. They didn't subject other people to their will. They succeeded from the inside out.

The people of these communities are historically known as the Sikhs. Sikh means student or seeker of truth. Today Sikhism has blossomed into a religion in its own right, with a greater community that includes more than 26 million people around the world, but it's significant to remember that it actually started as a revolution of consciousness; a movement of social and economic equality; of religious inclusion and tolerance; and a spiritual path to give people the tools to heal themselves, awaken themselves and create a better life for themselves and for those around them.

---

[1] Pronounced *Guroo Naanak*, we've maintained the traditional English spelling throughout these lectures. Guru Nanak, first Guru or Master in the Sikh Tradition. He lived from 1469-1539.

How did they do it? What were their secrets? In the midst of an incredibly oppressive society, what did they understand about human potential that allowed them to reinvent themselves—not through force or political pressure—but simply from the power of their own being?

Yogi Bhajan, Master of Kundalini Yoga and Siri Singh Sahib of *Sikh Dharma*, shared these secrets in his teachings about success, spirituality and prosperity. Here, for the first time, we have compiled a collection of Yogi Bhajan's lectures on how prosperity is a natural expression of the human spirit; how the soul and the Creator work in harmony with each other to create success in life on all levels; and how our own fears and limitations block us from living our destiny.

The essence of these teachings shows us that once we conquer our fears through meditation and access our intuition, there is no need to manipulate or hustle our way through life. What we need will come to us automatically, without our needing to ask for it. It is a perspective that does not avoid challenge, but welcomes it as an agent of growth and expansion. It is a perspective rooted in the belief that we are all part of One Creator, who works on our behalf when we stay connected to our spirit. But most of all, it is a perspective of personal responsibility—that to be human is to be successful, and to be successful requires that you share and that you uplift others. In this cycle of touching your own spirit, becoming successful and then uplifting other people, you become a force for peace, harmony and prosperity on the earth.

Yogi Bhajan was a unique being who learned, mastered and shared the ancient practices of Kundalini Yoga. In addition to being a yoga master, Yogi Bhajan was dedicated to *Sikh Dharma*, the Sikh way of life. With Kundalini Yoga, he gave people the tools to unlock their Infinite potential. Through *Sikh Dharma*, he shared a truly universal vision centered around using one's Infinite potential to build a world of peace, equality, grace, service, religious tolerance, respect for women and goodwill to all people. These teachings permeated every aspect of his own life, and he shared them in that same way. While teaching a Kundalini Yoga class, he would quote Guru Nanak or other Sikh Masters, or tell a story from Sikh history. When he spoke as the Siri Singh Sahib of *Sikh Dharma*, he would, in turn, reference Kundalini Yoga to illuminate the teachings of the Sikh Masters. In his teachings, these subjects worked together seamlessly and that is how he shared them.

You will see the same intermingling of teachings, stories and techniques from Kundalini Yoga and *Sikh Dharma* within this collection. We've included many wonderful meditations he gave over the years to develop the capacity for success. There are also sacred songs, called shabads, from the Sikh teachings that Yogi Bhajan encouraged people to practice. As the Siri Singh Sahib, he often talked about the *Shabad Guru* as the path of one who meditates on the enlightened words of the masters to awaken to one's own Infinite reality. For him, the *Shabad Guru* was integral to the practice of Kundalini Yoga because of the way it tempers the ego. The *Shabad Guru* gives a person something higher than themselves and their egos to relate to and merge with.

Yogi Bhajan was a visionary and the teachings he delivered transcend the time and space of his own lifetime. He was born to share a spiritual technology that was relevant to the future and the changing of the Ages. The dawning of the Age of Aquarius, the Mayan Calendar, the evolution of the human spirit—however you want to describe it—Yogi Bhajan saw the very real shift that humanity was about to navigate and believed that prosperity is one of the keys to success during the transition.

We hope that these lectures, meditations and shabads will help you awaken your own infinite potential for success and service to others. May you come to recognize and sense the true power you have as a human, and may you embrace that power with grace and reverence. Most of all, we pray that your own life will unfold into ever expanding cycles of ease, peace and contentment so that the future for you, your family and your community will be bright, blissful and beautiful. Sat Nam.

With Divine Light.

Yours humbly,

SS Ek Ong Kaar Kaur Khalsa
Creative Director, Sikh Dharma International

THE STORY OF HOW
I BECAME RICH

A student asked Yogi Bhajan the following question:
　　"Is giving an act of God?"

Yogi Bhajan replied, "No, no, no, no. Not at all. It is a perfectly selfish act. Have you heard about when I became rich? Listen to this. It is true. Verbatim, this is exactly true."

I taught a class at the East-West Cultural Center. And I did a wonderful job. There were three hundred and some dollars collected at class. I do not know exactly how much. But I definitely know one hundred fifty and some cents were given to me in an envelope as my fifty percent of that lecture. This is what they do. You go. They advertise you. You teach in that center. And whatever money comes in on that day, fifty percent is given to the lecturer and fifty percent goes to the center.

I did that. Then the director of the center takes the speaker out to dinner.

Now this lady, the director, was more spiritual, well-read with the scripture and much wiser than I was. I was very happy with her and she was extremely happy with me, because when she would talk scriptures, somewhere along the line, I'd give her the understanding of the scripture. I'm not very good with all this bookish knowledge but certain things I just know.

She said, "Today your lecture was so pleasing. I just want to take you to eat. Please come with me." She was just overwhelmingly joyful.

I said to her, "Well, there seems to be a storm behind the sunshine."

"What can it be?"

"We'll see."

When we came to the restaurant, on the side there was a pole. Standing beside the pole was a very beautiful, well-dressed black man. And he was saying, "I do not want to beg, and I don't want you to help me, but I have children. I have a life, and I have a family. I am selling these pencils. You can buy these pencils for any amount, because I am blind and can't see it. But I hope by the end of the day there will be a profit and I can take care of my family."

When I heard that I handed over my envelope to him and I took one pencil out. She saw me doing that and God, that divine woman became a living fire. She said, "What have you done? You know, that's what Indians do. You have encouraged beggary." She was so rude.

I said, "Ohhhhh!" That was my first experience, awakening the mind to encounter the bitchiness of an American woman. Up until then I was fine. I said, "What have I done?"

"You took one pencil for one hundred and fifty dollars. Do you know that you can get a truckload of them?"

"I don't need a truckload of pencils."

"Why did you take one pencil?"

"I want this one pencil to write my own fortune."

"And you paid one hundred and fifty dollars for it?"

"No. I paid much less. I paid nothing."

"I don't understand you. You don't like money. You don't love money."

I said, "I love money more than you like it. I love money. Don't worry about that. I just wanted this pencil to write my fortune. I paid the money you gave to me."

She said, "I can't believe it."

Meanwhile, we entered the restaurant. Then you know what she said? She said, "All right. I'll teach you something practical."

"Sure."

"I'm not going to pay for your dinner."

"Sure."

"That will show you what happens when you don't have money."

I said, "Sure. It's okay."

So I took my plate to the place where you pick up your salad, and you pick up this and that and I picked up everything I wanted to eat. I walked to the tables and the lady at the check-out counter said, "Thank you, sir." She never says that. I just went up there, took the things off the tray, and put them on the table. We were about three or four people and when the director came, the counter clerk told her, "Thank you, ma'am. You can pass."

She said, "Who paid for it?"

The clerk said, "It is all paid for."

So, she felt a little small and she came and sat down next to me me. Meanwhile, the counter girl came and brought sixty-some dollars and gave it to me. Imagine. I didn't have a pocket. I didn't have a dollar. I didn't have a penny. She told me that she isn't going to pay and I said to the counter clerk, "Give it to her."

The clerk said, "No, no. It is for you, sir. It is for you."

"Why for me?"

"There was a student of yours sitting here. He left me with a hundred dollars and he said, 'My teacher is coming. All the people with him should be paid for, and the balance given to him.' So I am just doing what he said."

I looked at the director. I said, "You didn't pay for it?"

"No."

"You got paid for, too?"

"Yes."

I said, "See how God works?" And I pulled out ten dollars and I gave it to the waitress.

She said, "O my God. Thank you. Thank you. Thank you."

And I gave the director the fifty-some remaining dollars.

She asked me, "What for? I don't understand. You seem so happy."

I said, "Today, my Guru and my God have made me a giver. Before this, I was a taker. I was at your mercy. And when you tested it, Guru came through. He saved me at the last minute. I am very mad at Him for that. But because he always does it, I am very grateful. I have seen my Guru. I have seen Him in action. I am grateful."

CHAPTER ONE

LIKE THE FRAGRANCE
OF A ROSE

The subject we are discussing is very serious and extremely simple. What should you do to bring prosperity to your life?

Prosperity doesn't mean that you will have wealth, health and happiness. The best way to explain prosperity is to say it is like a rosebud when it flowers and opens up, and shares its fragrance. That's the moment, which lasts a few days, when a rose flower is prosperous. When a man or woman is prosperous, it is the fragrance of security, grace, depth, character and truthfulness that a person can share. Like a candle emits light, a human emits prosperity.

We misunderstand prosperity. If somebody is rich, has a big house, has money, has a business, is successful and all that, we say he is prosperous.

Once, there was a very prosperous man. I met him in California. He told me he has forty thousand acres of orchards—almonds, walnuts, this and that. He even took me in a jeep to tour his territory. When we came back home, we sat down. We were sweating and I said, "You have forty thousand acres of land, right? By deed."

He said, "Yes, that's true."

"But how many acres belong to you?"

"All of them."

"What is under the bank loan?"

"All of it."

"So you work hard, you grow these things and you work it out. Then you pay the installment to the bank, you pay the labor, you pay the insurance, you pay the workmen compensation, and all that. Then what exactly do you save?"

He said, "Nothing."

"So why you do this?"

"One day I hope it will cover me and I will cover it."

This is how your life is. You come here, you educate yourself, you graduate. Then you work hard in life. You work during the day and sometimes you work two jobs, sometimes one job. Sometimes you think you are very wonderful, very powerful. You want your freedom. You want your thoughts. You want your expression. You want your sex. You want your partner. You want your home. You make a lot of decisions. But in reality, after a while, when all that glitter goes away, you start realizing you were on the wrong track. As long as you work hard, you plan and you push, there is no fun. But there is a state of mind that we are going to talk about today. It's called the way to prosperity where things come to you.

Things come to you. You can understand when you were born, your security was taken care of by your parents. You were brought up by your parents and every relative would kiss you, hug you and take care of you. The moment you lost your innocence, you had to hustle for yourself. When you grew up, then your mother expected something but you couldn't do it so there was a fight. Your father expected something but you couldn't do it so there was a fight. Your brothers started going after each other's jugular. Your sisters wanted their own thing. And that bouquet of flowers you had when you were born became scattered straw.

Then you fell in love with somebody. "Oh! She loves me. Oh! I love her." And it is funny, after a couple of years, that wears out. "Oh, I didn't marry you for that. I didn't like you like that." And you are on each other's backs.

What is it that makes us do this? There must be some reason that everybody does it—the question is why. It is because nobody is mature enough to take responsibility for their life. Nobody has a meditative mind to be intuitive to find out that they are on the wrong track.

When two trains are on the wrong track, they can collide head on. That's why people have their flow totally blocked up and dammed up. Once in a while they let loose and then there is no joy left in life. It is a misunderstanding on the part of a human. They act like animals. They think they can fight and get what they want. That's why you feel that the majority of people are rude. They do not know how to compromise. They do not know how to be nice.

These days, when you talk to people, they say, "Well, my mother did this to me … My father did this to me … My neighbor did it to me … My uncle did it to me," as if they only have other people to blame and that's it. But whatever your father, mother, uncle or neighbor did, now you are you. You have to be you. And the greatest tragedy of this time is that we all are trying to find God outside of us. So there are hundreds and thousands of organizations where people pray and pray. They say, "Pray." Pray for everybody and pray to God. Nobody knows what kind of prayer they are doing. Whether they are doing prayer or they are preying on people—nobody knows. They think God Almighty is somewhere in the seventh heaven and we are here and we have to try to find Him.

The reality is that God is inside. Nobody is even responsible enough to acknowledge it. God is within me. Therefore, I have to act like God's existence. Nobody wants to act like God's creature.

Somebody is proud of his richness. Somebody is proud of his beauty. Somebody is proud of his environments. Some people are very proud of their political power. They want to convince others that they are the best on the earth. That's a human weakness. One of the most sociological and psychological weaknesses of humans is that they want to impress others. Yet, once they start impressing themselves, it's Nirvana. They are redeemed. They are free. They get whatever they want.

Because once the candle is lit, there is no dearth of moths. They will come. Once a man is illumined, there is no dearth of *maya*[2]. It will come.

Life is not set up for us to suffer. Happiness is the birthright of the person, provided you feel—at least a little honestly— that God is within you. God is *prana*[3], life. If God is not life, then what is God? Dead? There is no dead God. God is alive. His existence is alive. As long as you live, there is a God for you. The moment you don't live, forget it.

We have theories. We have ideas and we have philosophies. We want to deal with life as we want it. But actually, what is life? We are on sale. We don't go to an interview naturally. We want to change. We want to look good. We want to feel good. We want to make another person feel we are good. All right, you feel very good and attractive and you go about and things happen. But what about your faculty? Your faculty has an identity. Who is going to work? You can fix up a beautiful zebra to look like an Arabian horse, but who is going to walk it? Can a giraffe become an elephant? How much makeup can you use? How much can you cover yourself? How many methods do you use to look pretty and beautiful and loving and all that, when there is no juice in you? When your mind—your own mind—cannot stand you? People say, "I don't know." You know, these are the craziest people. I have seen people who are very educated who come to me and say, "I can't. I can't do it. I can't."

"Why not? Have you tried?"

"No, I can't do it."

They are scared like a crow. What have we become? Born in the image of God as human, we have become toys to be sold to a Christmas shopping list. Everybody is crazy. Shop, shop, shop. Gift, gift, gift. Gift what? Gift yourself peace and tranquility. Gift yourself grace and honor. Gift yourself a few moments of prayer to purify yourself. But that's not what happens.

---

[2] *Maya* refers to the material and sensual world.
[3] *Prana* is a yogic term referring to the breath of life.

Before Christ, there used to be something called the "White Holidays." For ten days, the Romans would never fight, never conquer anybody, and never attack. Those people were not Christians, they were Heathens. But for those ten days they would sit and meditate. They would not move. And Jesus Christ's birthday—Jesus was born on the twenty-fifth of August—was shifted to the twenty-fifth of December to suit the Roman White Holidays. That's how honest we are to him. First we put him on a cross, then we shift his birthday because it suits us. It is amazing how men, people, countries and nations have shifted things to their convenience.

It is a funny thing how countries change—how people change. The Czar of Russia was very mad one day. He said, "I want to adopt a religion that will work for me."

So he sent five people all over the world. They went to India. They went everywhere and when they came back, they said, "Well, the Indians are very funny."

The Czar said, "Why?"

"They accept everything but they accept nothing."

He said, "No. That's not for us. What else?"

"There are Jews."

"What is the problem with them?"

"They are great, wise, and perfect. But, they don't eat pork."

The Czar said, "That's not for us. We hunt boars."

"Well, there is another thing. Christianity."

"What about that?"

"They are all right. They eat everything. They accept everything and they love God."

He said, "What about Islam?"

"It's the same problem. They don't eat pork."

He said, "Let us all be Christian."

That's how it was decided.

> *If it is considered possible that man is born out of the will of God and in the image of God; that man is divine and that he has no duality; and that a divine person has no needs, then all that there is will come to that person.*

Man wants concessions. Man wants concessions with his body, with his health, with his environments and with his friends. Something easy—something that just comes to him out of nothing. Because man has never recognized that man has never come out of nothing. Man is born out of the will of God, but has not recognized the basic value of being a human. They are still little kids getting their diapers changed. When they grow up as elders, it is the same continuous thing. Somebody has to do something for somebody. And there is this constant devaluation of life, "We come from nothing, we are nothing. How can we know we can be something?" As the very evaluation of man, this thought, process makes people non-prosperous.

If it is considered possible that man is born out of the will of God and in the image of God; that man is divine and that he has no duality; and that a divine person has no needs, then all of what there is will come to that person. At the right time, the right things will appear. There is no reason for suffering and for being nasty.

Somebody once saw a bunch of money. His first thought was, "I will pick it up." His second thought was, "It doesn't belong to me." Third, he picked it up and took it to a place to return it and said, "Well, this money doesn't belong to me. I found it on the road. Maybe somebody will claim it."

The guy looked at him and said, "Hey, why you are returning it? It is 50-50."

The first man said, "What is 50-50?"

"It is a lot of money. You can keep half and I can keep half and we end the matter."

"No. You can keep the half or have the whole, I am not concerned. I have to answer to my consciousness. You have to answer yours."

While going home, he stopped at a shop and got a ticket, one lotto ticket. He went home and there were thirty-two million dollars announced for that lottery ticket. He went back to see the second guy and he said, "Did you return it?"

"Yes."

"Has somebody claimed it?"

"Yes"

The first man said. "Good."

The second guy said, "But there is a $2,000 reward for you. Sign for it and take it."

That's how God works—through miracles. Your life is not yours. It depends upon your purity of consciousness, how compassionate, kind and caring you are.

If you concern yourself with how much muscle you have got and how many people you can punch; how many people you can cheat and how sharp you are; how you cut corners with everybody, and how stupid you are to use other people for your purposes—fine. Enjoy yourself. You are stupid. That's not the bright side of the human. That's the dark side of the devil. Life is not given to you for those kinds of dirty games.

And then you wear very good clothes, makeup and hairdo, and this and that. Polish and cream. A 60-year-old man lying down like an idiot, trying to remove his wrinkles and get his skin burnt. Who can tell you what to do? Nobody. The church lives off your money. The synagogue lives off your money. All these swamis and yogis live off your money. You are the Gods, totally blind and stupid Gods.

Only Santa Claus knows you. He promises his sack of gifts and you go berserk spending billions of dollars. You see what a commercial way of life it is? Before it was Santa Claus, it was Saint Nicholas in northern Germany. Somebody in New York made too many long socks and they didn't sell. So the next year he made up a story of Santa Claus. You know people who did not even have chimneys in their house still bought gifts?

And look what happened to the Christmas tree. The Christmas tree is the evergreen tree that never dies in winter. Once I sent a card to everyone I knew. It said, "The Christmas tree asked God, 'Why did you name me so? Every year they cut me down. They don't let me grow.'" What do you do to this pure sign of life and livelihood when there is snow? You cut it down, bring it home and then throw it away. You have satisfied your ego.

The Christmas tree tradition, as I knew it, used to be that in front of the house, there would be a big tree. At night they would put all the presents under it and in the morning the children would go and play, run, sing and then go under the tree. It used to be a big tree and not a little teeny, tiny nonsense that you buy for $150. Now they have a cup for it to stand in. This is how things go from normal to abnormal and from abnormal to nothing. What we don't have is character. We do not have commitment. We walk empty in this life.

We are looking for something. Life has a very serious problem. I want to tell you what life is all about. Life has a constant action and reaction that you cannot stop. Your inner anger and your outer fear cannot let you be anything but a reactionary, everlasting nuisance. You do not develop maturity and common ground with everybody in the world.

If you cannot see God in all, you cannot see God at all. Everything is God—everything from a stone to a mountain.

So this is the life we have come to deal with. There is a way to prosperity. If the mind is clear, if the subconscious is not blocked, if you unconsciously live a conscious life, you can never be poor. Where there is a magnet, things will fly to it. The mastermind, the Great Mind, knows your needs. You don't have to yell and scream, "Help, God!" God is inside. He manufactured you. He sent you here. He gave you features and facets. He gave you all the environments you need. You simply do not accept it. I am just explaining it to you.

The fact is, someday, somewhere, just be yourself. Let everything go. That day you will find you are you. Oh God! The very joy of you being you is the most precious joy. It will take away all your suffering. It will take away your pain. You will find you within you—there is nothing more than that.

Look, I found myself within myself, and I found you as a plus. You all came. I came. We have met. We are acting to reach a faculty of life that is consolidated, that is ours. We are reaching for a life that does not give any false hope because it has no lies in it. It does not create a picture or a fantasy that is untrue. It is a life of reality that tells you that you are you. Yet, you don't want to listen to it.

You have never tried to listen to the fact from your own self that you are you. And you do not understand the fact that you have a very precious, fair life. It has come to you as a gift. Life is demanding. Don't drift. Be something.

You think that money does everything—that if we have money, we are free? A lot of people meet me. They say, "We have money, we can take care of everything." What everything? If you have a cold, with $2,000 on your face you can't get rid of it. Who do you think you are kidding? All the money in the world cannot get rid of heart disease. Tons of money cannot take care of your liver. But daikon radish can.

Money is a medium. It's not the ultimate solution. Life has to come through the purity of wisdom and the mutuality of relationships. I am me and you are you. Somewhere we have to meet and that mutual ground is called wisdom. Wisdom is when two flexibilities meet and decide a situation. Then there is happiness. But when you push your own buttons, and somebody else pushes their buttons, then there is a war.

So let us meditate[4] and see if our mind can be cleansed. And if we can reach the state of mind where we can feel something. Why do we meditate? We have one thousand thoughts per wink of the eye. Millions, zillions of thoughts. Out of that, a few become feelings and then

---

[4] In the meditation section: What You Should Do To Bring Prosperity To Your Life. © The Teachings of Yogi Bhajan, December 26, 1997.

feelings become emotions and then emotions become desires. It's a constant cycle. But we need some space. When the consciousness gets filled with thoughts and desires, it starts unloading from the subconscious. And then you have nightmares. Then you are Mr. Nobody.

You must know you have an unlimited reserve of energy. Once you invoke your energy, there is nothing that is small in you. All the environments start flying towards you. It's beautiful.

May I know myself to know my Maker. May I know myself to know my universe. May I know myself to know the beauty and bounty and purpose and prosperity of my life. Without personal knowledge there is no knowledge. Without personal knowledge there is no width, height or horizon. I pray to Thee, oh Lord, as you are within me, to give me tranquility and peace between me and myself so that I can know myself on the way of prosperity. I pray in thy name. Sat Nam.

Money is a medium.

It's not the ultimate solution.

CHAPTER TWO

THE PURPOSE OF LIFE

Virtues are virtues and wishes are wishes. Every human being wants to have more virtues, and wishes for much more than virtues. The question is how to have it. The question is not whether you can go to a restaurant and have a 35- or 36-course meal and enjoy the evening. That is possible. The question is whether your stomach can take it or not—that is the question.

The question is not how you live. You have the right to live as you want. That is not the question. The question is, are you living within your understanding of who you are? That is the question. The question is not whether you are virtuous or wishful, the question is, have you understood your commitment and the depth of your commitment?

What does it mean to live a full life? A full life is when a man has both his commitment and an understanding of his commitment—and even death cannot change it. Guru Nanak had a commitment. Death couldn't change it. Jesus Christ had a commitment. Death couldn't change it. Moses had a commitment. For 40 years he carried the commandments through the desert without any change.

When man has spiritual ecstasy and elevation, forget about temptation, even death can't change him. Such a person creates a legacy. The person dies and the legacy lives. That is the only beauty granted to a human being.

How many times you get married; how many times you become unmarried. How many times you are a Sikh; how many times you are not a Sikh. How many times you are human; how many times you are not human. You know 500 lifetimes in the past; you know 5,000 lifetimes in the future. You can make rain; you can not make rain. You can produce gold; you can lose gold. All that is nonsense—it is totally material. It does not matter how material or non-material you are. What matters is whether death can lose you or you can lose death. It is true that Jesu the Carpenter set the renaissance. Gautam Buddha the Prince set the renaissance. Nanak the Guru set the renaissance. Mohammed the Hazarat set the renaissance. Did death eliminate them? No. Death is as life is.

ਜੋ ਉਪਜਿਓ ਸੋ ਬਿਨਸਿ ਹੈ ਪਰੋ ਆਜੁ ਕੈ ਕਾਲਿ

Jo upji-o so binas hai paro aaj kai kaal.

Whatever has been created shall be destroyed;
everyone shall perish, today or tomorrow.

— Guru Teg Bahadur[5], *Siri Guru Granth Sahib,* page 1429, line 4

Whosoever has to be born shall die. The purpose of life is when death cannot kill you. Man can kill a man. Poison can kill a man. Disease can kill a man. The will of God can kill a man. God can kill a man. It is all true—I have no dispute with it. But is it true? No. Is Jesus dead? No. Is Guru Nanak dead? No. Is Buddha dead? No. When we are alive we do not know whether we will live forever or not. When a mortal is mortal, he does not know whether he can become immortal. But when death takes its toll, a mortal can become immortal, then that immortality becomes the legacy. And that is the purpose of life.

Why don't we burn people once they have died? We put them in graves. We carve their memory into the stones. Once in a while, some relatives go and put flowers on the grave. Sometimes when we are young lovers, we go someplace and write our names on mountains and on stones. Sometimes when we sit together, we carve our names on the trees—first the initials and then a lot of hugs and crosses.

It is the distinct nature of the soul that it comes on the earth to live forever by merging into the Creator that we call God. It has a price. That price we have to pay is taught as a science called *dharma*—whichever *dharma* it is. The art of living is what the dictates are. Every religion is beautiful. There is no dispute that religions are beautiful. You can convert to any religion; you can change to any form and shape. But have you understood reality or not? That matters. You are a human. Have you understood what a human is? That matters.

Whether you are a good person, a bad person, a rich person, a poor person, a religious person or a fake doesn't mean a thing. Why do we say, "God, save us from anger, greed, attachment, pride and lust"? Because these are the five senses that make a human being insane.

These five powers can be used properly. When you are angry either you have no control over your anger, or you can drive your anger towards your excellence and your purity—you can become God. What about Jesus? He went to school. The kids beat him up. "You are a bastard," they said. He came home and asked his mother, "Am I a bastard?" She said, "No. An angel came to me, and told me you are by the will of the Divine." "Who is my father?" She

---
[5] Guru Teg Bahadur, Ninth Guru or Master in the Sikh Tradition. He lived from 1621-1675.

said, "He is in the heavens." That's it. The kid stuck with it. The king told him, "Just change your statement." He said, "No, my father is the real king. I am in His kingdom not in yours." The poor Roman general begged him. "Please don't be so spaced out. Just make a little amends."

Then there was Guru Arjan. "Guru Arjan Partakh Har." Personified God. They asked him to sit on a hot plate.[6] "We will put hot sand on you and roast you like a potato." He sat. The Muslim saint Mian Mir said, "What is going on? If you don't want to do something, I will cool it for you." Guru Arjan said, "No. Somebody in human form who believes in me will sit on the hot plate in the future. I am just leading the way."

It doesn't matter if you are a Sikh or not. A Sikh is one who learns. If you are not learned, you are not learning. Then nothing shall work. If you are a Muslim, and you are not humble, then you cannot learn to be a Muslim. If you are a Buddhist and you do not have the wisdom to see God in all, then you are a baboon joker. If you are a Christian and cannot face crisis, then you better shut up. You don't know what a Christian is. Even in the Native American religion, if a man is not in a position to fight with a grizzly bear or a leopard or a lion, it is not considered brave.

A man who is not a hero with a soul is not a man. He is a statue. You wind him up. He works. This idiot dresses up, goes out the whole day, hassles, sweats, lies, plays games, fingers this, nails that, does this and comes back home—for just one smile on the face of his wife. This beggar looks around for acceptance. Can you believe what a shallow attribute of life it is?

Somebody once got very mad at me. My staff told me, "This guy is very mad at you."

"What do you want me to do? He is mad. He is a mad man. What should I do?"

"We don't want him to be mad at you."

"If you don't want him to be mad at me, it is very simple. Take 108 white roses. What is the bill?" In those days they were cheap. About 35, 40 dollars. "Send the roses to him."

So she sent them.

I said, "Write this note. May the whiteness of the roses and the fragrance uplift your spirit, and may the kindness in your heart forgive me. I cannot bear that you are mad at me for nothing. But if it is for something, still it is worthwhile not to be mad."

I said, "Write down this note and give it to him."

Five Cs [7]

Caliber
will make you deliver.

Character
will sustain you.

Consciousness
will carry you.

Courage
will bring you honor.

Commitment
will bring you trust.

---

[6] Guru Arjan Dev ji, Fifth Guru, or Master in the Sikh tradition. He lived from 1563-1606. Through a series of political intrigues, the sovereignty of Guru Arjan and his people was challenged by the Mughal Emperor Jahangir. To protect the independence of the community, Guru Arjan allowed himself to be tortured. He was chained to a hot metal plate while his captors poured burning sand on his body. It is said Guru Arjan smiled during the torture, seeing the hand of the Divine behind it. After five days and nights, Guru Arjan was permitted to bathe in a nearby river. He dove into the water and dissolved into Light. His physical body was never seen again.

[7] © The Teachings of Yogi Bhajan, September 3, 1996

Two long, typed pages came back. "I was not mad." What a lie. He was. "I was not mad. It was a misunderstanding. Please forgive me." I laughed at what $40 can do.

You can do whatever you want, but when it is a matter of fate and destiny, then let it be. No interference is required. Between man and God there are two paths: the path of fate and the path of destiny. Those who will give distance to their destiny shall fall into the path of fate. When you walk on the path of fate, you may feel very happy and be an egomaniac, but when the fatal moment comes, you will be lost again. When you walk on the path of destiny, it doesn't matter what distance you cover. When the fatal blow of death comes, you shall be liberated. That is all—that is the difference.

All this chanting, the religious rituals and religious ceremonies—the whole life we live—is for that last moment. Was I true to my *dharma*, or was I not? There comes a moment before death when you are judged in the trinity of you, your destiny, and your fate. And that judgment is your decision—nobody else's.

Doing yoga practices and doing rituals—all of it—is to remind and re-remind us to develop that habit. This is why prayer is powerful. When you are helpless, when you are absolutely weak, you are gone, you are nothing, you are hanging with this little thread between life and death, all of what you have done in your life either reminds you of God or not.

Take a girl and a boy. They make love, they get married, spend millions of dollars, feed 60,000 people, have the press carry the story. Then go on the honeymoon and come back. If the man is impotent, how long will their marriage last? It won't.

It is that impotency of karma that takes *dharma* away from you. You start the sequence that creates the consequences and, finally, you lose the game. Why? Because you do not have your intuition under your control. The divine guidance is not there. Whenever a man is guided by his ego, insult in the court of God is guaranteed. God's kingdom has a direct animosity with ego.

Ego and divinity will never walk together. When you burn a candle, the darkness will go away. Put out the candle and the darkness will come back. There are no two opinions.

Why do we need intuition? We need it in every moment. Why? Because I want to know. And if I don't know, I have to hustle. And then I waste all that precious life in hustling.

When I came to America, I didn't know anything. I didn't know what a boulevard was or a turnpike. When I heard the word "freeway," I said, "What? Everywhere else you pay for the ticket. This thing you go on for free?" That is how freeway sounds.

One person I knew here thought I was a freeloader. Somehow the husband and wife started yelling and screaming over it. I understood.

One evening, we were sitting together eating food in his house. He said, "Well, Bhajan, you are not learning anything about America."

"What do I have to learn?"

"Start driving a car. Learn how to drive a car."

"I know how to drive a car. Why do I have to learn how to drive a car? I know how to drive a car."

"Oh no. It is not India."

"What are you saying? I know I am in America."

"People here drive on the right."

I said, "There they drive on the left. Here you drive on the right. If you do not know how to drive from left to right, right to left, what kind of man are you? I know how to drive on the right. I know how to drive. But I am not going to drive."

"Why not?"

"I am not going to drive. Period."

"Well, how will you get around?"

"I don't know."

"Who will drive you?"

"You. What kind of brother are you if you can't drive me?"

He said, "You are not listening. Be practical."

"Be practical? What do you mean?"

"It is a necessity in Los Angeles. One should have his own car."

I said, "What else?"

"I want you to drive."

"What else?"

"Then you can go where you want to go."

"Well, listen to me. I will go where I want to go, but I am not going to drive."

"Why not? Why are you so against it?"

I said, "One thing I want to tell you. When I was in India, I worked for the government of India. I had a car, I had a driver, I had a cleaner, I had a mechanic and I had an orderly. Now I am going to serve God and I am going to drive? Are you an idiot?"

He said, "One doesn't have anything to do with the other."

I said, "I don't want to be demoted. I don't want to drive."

"Who will drive you?"

"Whosoever shall drive me shall be prosperous, regal and gracious. It's a privilege."

"Ah forget this yogi bullshit. Nonsense, nonsense, nonsense."

I said, "What? What did you say? What is bullshit?" I didn't know the meaning of the word bullshit.

"The dirt," he said. He was very angry. "You are crazy,"

I said, "Okay, let's not fight with each other. Let's leave it here. We will discuss it tomorrow."

He said, "Okay." So we departed and went on our way.

In the morning, he was going to the office and I was ready with my little Air France bag. He said, "Are you leaving?"

I said, "Yeah."

"Why?"

"I'm a guest where I'm not welcome."

"But you are my brother."

"Well that's okay, but it's not true that brothers are welcome all the time."

"Where are you going?"

"I don't know."

"Well, heck, get in my car. I will drive you where you want."

"No. I am not sitting in your car and you are not driving me today."

"Well, where are you going?"

I said, "I don't know. Why should I tell you where I am going?"

So we started moving. I walked on my pathway. He started driving in his Cadillac. We came from Baldwin Hill down a little bit, about 100 to 200 yards and he said, "Don't torture me. I can't stand it. Get in the car."

"I said, no and I meant no."

"You are crazy."

"Yeah, you told me last night. This is the second time. Don't tell me a third time or I am going to tell you that you are crazy and you will be. Be afraid of it. I really mean business."

"Who is going to drive you?"

"A car will come that is better than your car, and the driver will be better than you."

"This is a Cadillac."

"Something has to be a little better than this to pick me up."

"Stop this. You are confusing me."

I said, "No, I am not. I am speaking truthfully."

We turned the corner and here comes a Continental. And the guy who is driving yells, "Oh Yogiji, Yogi Bahan, Yogi Bahan." I used to be Yogi Bahan in those days.

I said, "Hey look at that. It's whiter. It's bigger and it's being driven by a chauffeur. Do you get the message?"

He said, "But where are you going?"

"I don't know. But wherever I go, I will call you tonight. I will let you know."

The driver stopped the car, and opened the door. I got in and said, "See?" And we drove away. I never went back to his house to live again.

I called him in the evening. I said, "I have a house. I have food here and there are two attendants with me. I don't know where it is, but I can tell you the telephone number. It is somewhere in Hollywood."

"Who you are living with?"

"This guy I told you about. He is a health restaurant man. It is his car. He sent it for me."

"He got a house for you?"

"Yes. It's paid for. It is completely rented and paid for. Everything is set here."

"What are you going to do there?"

I said, "Nothing. I told you. I don't do a thing. Didn't you hear? I mean, it's a simple word in English. You don't understand. It is called 'nothing.'"

"Who does everything for you?"

"Somebody up there."

"Would you like to introduce me to him sometime?"

I said, "Look, brother. I was in your house. You should have learned then. Now the time is over. There are certain things I know. There are certain things you know. What you know, I don't know. And what I know, you don't know. You never asked me. I didn't push myself on you. But, as long as I live in the United States, there will always be somebody to drive me. I just wanted to tell you that. And that car will always be bigger than yours."

And it is true.

Another time something similar happened. My limousine was a diesel. It made a lot of noise when it started, like a cracked up thing. One day my man, my protocol officer, said, "I hate this car. It makes so much noise."

"Well, we didn't ask for it. God gave it to us. Let's drive it. It wakes up. It makes a lot of mess."

"If I can get a car that is not a diesel like this, I'll get it right now."

"So be it."

So we went to meet someone. We were having a different conversation and my protocol officer mentioned his anger over the car. The person we were meeting with said, "Wait a minute. That's Yogiji's car. It has been sitting here with me for the last ten years. I brought it from Germany. It is absolutely new. It's yours." He fixed it up and gave us the key.

I said, "See? Now you can drive this car. It's not a diesel."

I asked my staff why I hadn't gotten that car before and they said, "You don't have an account for the insurance." Somebody has given a car—an absolutely good car—but there is no allotment for extra insurance. They even asked me, "Are you going to pay the insurance or will somebody else?"

I said, "Don't worry. Somebody will pay it. We didn't buy the car. Why should we pay for the insurance? Let it sit. When there is insurance, then we will drive it."

You can call this attitude fatalistic. I call it intuitive. The hand of Guru Ram Das[7] is so blessed—it's a strength. The miracle is when God starts taking care of you and you stop taking care of your own BS—pardon the expression—your "Beautiful Service," which you do to yourself because of your ego.

It is not true that I have never been insulted. It is not true that I have never been dragged down. It is not true that I have never had painful moments. It is not true that I have never gone to the hospital. What is true is that there is nothing bad in the world that I have not gone through, but I have gone through it in the ecstasy of prayer.

A headache is a headache. Tylenol doesn't remove the cause of the headache. But you don't feel it. That is spiritual. When you don't feel the pangs of negativity, anger, commotion and vengeance, then you are saintly. That is the beauty of the Sixth Chakra. That is the beauty of the Third Eye. That is the beauty of the human. Not that you look like a human, but live like an emotional idiot. That is not beauty. That is survival.

You have a beautiful, double king-sized bed with a satin back, canopy, the whole thing. The guy who is lying there can't sleep—he is suffering with insomnia. What is the use? Then you see somebody else who has a brick under his head, and his snore sounds like a rattlesnake that you can hear far away in the distance.

The question is not whether you are a man or not. The question is whether you have endurance or not. The question is not whether you are religious or not. The question is, do you have perpetual endurance or not? That's the question. Are you even enough to survive against all odds? There is only one way to do it. You must have your own intuition and your spirit must talk to you.

---

[7] Guru Ram Das ji (1534-1581) was the fourth Master in the Sikh tradition. It is said that the throne of *Raj Yog*—of Royal Yoga—was bestowed on him. Yogi Bhajan had a special connection to Guru Ram Das throughout his life.

Somebody has sent me flowers. I'm the cause. Somebody has sent flowers for me, but it is a fact that they will go on the altar. You send flowers to anybody else and they won't go on the altar. You will get a letter of appreciation. I won't write an appreciation letter. That is the difference between finite and Infinity. They will go on the altar, we will pray and ask God, whosoever has decorated your altar, decorate that being. That is called God's way. The rest is human.

Intuition. The word has a prefix. It will cut across human rational logic and set you on faith.

*The miracle is when God
starts taking care of you
and you stop taking care
of your own BS.*

CHAPTER THREE

INNER CALLING, OUTER CALLING

Once a man said to a sage, "My lord, I am not very happy."
The saint replied, "It's just karma."

"My lord, what is karma?"

"You are not happy. That's karma."

He looked around and he said, "Perhaps you have not understood my question."

The sage said, "What is your question?"

"I am not happy."

"I told you, it's karma."

"How can I get rid of karma?"

"Go somewhere and get *dharma*."

He said, "My lord, I have not understood what *dharma* is."

The sage said, "*Dharma* is when you answer your inner calling."

"What is my inner calling?"

"It's a very subtle thing called consciousness."

The man said, "That's right. There is a sound—a very meek, beautiful little thing in me that talks to me. But it's too weak. I don't want to hear it."

The sage said, "That is consciousness. There is not one person who can live and whose conscience doesn't speak."

"My lord, my consciousness speaks, but I always ignore it."

"That's ego. Ego, my son, is only for local time and space. But you are not time and space—you are *Atman* (the soul). You are not born and you do not die. You come from the Infinite, from the Unknown. You pass through the known, to merge into the Unknown. If you want to merge into the Unknown, you have to have *dharma*."

"My lord, I have heard that there is a consciousness and I have to hear it. But is there any way that I can understand it in my language?"

The sage said, "My son, there is a thing called 'Calling.'"

"Yes."

"Do people speak to you? Do they ask you something?"

"Yes."

"That is calling. From a stone, from a tree, from a person, from a bird. All that is God. When anything calls on you, answer it with strength and grace—that is *dharma*."

He went home and his wife said, "Where were you?"

"I went to see a saint."

"Why did you go to see a saint?"

"I had a calling that I should go and see some man of God, so I went."

"You forgot that I am your wife? I have a calling, too. That work is not done."

"That is true, but I had to go."

"Do you understand my calling?"

"Yes."

Then the son said, "You promised me that you would go with me to a certain place, but you didn't show up. What kind of father do I have?"

So one thing led to another. Everything started calling him, asking him to answer, asking him to question, asking him to do things. He dealt with it for a while then went to the man of God again and said, "Lord, I went there and I don't know which calling is which. You said there is a calling. There was an inner calling so I came here. And now there is an inner calling to run, so I have come here again. Because everybody is calling on me and I do not know what to do."

The man of God said, "When people call, answer them with a smile. Raise their consciousness. That act will, in turn, raise your consciousness many times, manifold."

The man went back home. His wife said, "You were missing again."

"Oh my dear girl, it was such a lofty situation. I went there to see when I can bring you there, too."

"What was it like?"

"I had such an experience. I felt like . . ." And he put the whole fantasy into it.

She said, "Let us go now."

"No, no, no, no, no. I have to do something for my son. Let me do that." So he went to his son.

The son said, "Why are you so late?"

When you carry your
goodness, your grace, your
brightness, your light, your
bounty, your beauty—
you carry it on and carry it on
and carry it on.

"I had such a fancy feeling. I met a man. I was uplifted. I was appreciated. You don't understand, my son."

"Papa, can I go, too?"

So a few days later he took his whole family. The man of God smiled.

The man said, "My lord, you have smiled."

The sage said, "This is called Sadh Sangat—congregation. If it is imagined, it is uplifted. You have all come and many more will come with this inner feeling. In return, you will find there is something better in you, higher in you and more pure in you. And that is redemption, that is resurrection."

Water has to resurrect from the very chest of the ocean to the sky and then it has to travel back and kiss the gold peaks of the mountain to become rain. It must shower like the mercy of a man and must flow through the heart of the land, to reach its goal, to cover the distance into destiny. That's the process of life.

Every human being needs loftiness, exaltedness, self-confidence, and appreciation to be grateful that we are alive at this moment and we are alive together. It's like stars in the sky on the same night. Some are big. Some are small. Some are shining. Some come late. Some come earlier. But in the brim of night, all are lit on their axle. On their orbit, they exist. That is the condition of every human.

The comparative study of how to learn, to grow and to be is *dharma*. To compete, compare and be confused is a low-grade karma. We are all born. There are a lot of people who are rich. There are a lot of people who are wise. There are a lot of people who are powerful. There are a lot of people who are greatly unique. Are they fulfilled?

Go to a rich person—a very rich person. When you ask him for money, he'll say, "Ahh, you have come at the wrong time. We just invested yesterday."

Go to a talented person and just say, "I have come to learn something."

He'll say, "This is the time for sleep. I'll see you later."

If a human cannot extend himself or herself, that person cannot be redeemed. It is the light that must redeem itself by emitting, being radiant and reaching out.

There was once a saint who was very, very ill. He couldn't open his eyes. He was not even in a position to crawl. His disciples took him on their shoulders in a very decorated way, and carried him from village to village, from place to place. They went everywhere. They carried him and carried him to the yonderlands. There was a great collection of people and there were many gatherings. They prayed and they chanted and they blessed everybody. Finally, after three or four years, they returned home. In a feeble voice the saint said,

"Now you are all liberated. You are all saints. My time has come and I shall be gone."

The great man died. They did all the ceremonies and they read his will in which he said,

"I was very feeble, weak and unable to participate in all the holy pilgrimages, but you carried me. As you carried me, you have carried God in your hearts and grace in your heads. Keep on going."

And thus, afterwards, they did not stop. They all traveled to the yonderlands and they sang and they chanted and they blessed. Finally they realized they were just like their master. This is called the cycle of consciousness. When you carry your goodness, your grace, your brightness, your light, your bounty, your beauty—and you carry it on and carry it on and carry it on.

In the Age of Aquarius[8], the *dharma* of a person shall be to reach out. Reach out to help. Reach out to share smiles. Reach out to hear each other. Reach out to every person without judgment. It should be a quantum leap in the consciousness where a person will honor himself. It is my personal honor that I am a saint. It is my personal grace that I am a sage. It is my personal victory that I am a human. It is my personal joy that I am grateful and fulfilled. Everything is personal. Everything is shared and every person will try one's best.

You who are born in this time and in this moment, at this *desh* (space), and at this *kaal* (time) have a purpose in life. If you have a purpose in life and you don't have a projection[9] in life, you are losing something big. It is your *dharma* that you, through karma yoga, will serve anybody and everybody without discrimination. Thus you will cleanse yourself of your karma and you will be enlightened in the grace and happiness of your accomplishments. You are here now. None of us has features like each other. We are different in size, weight, shape and in caliber. Even in consciousness, even in development, we have come from different backgrounds. We have different experiences. We have different ideas. With all that, we are one because we are here. We are now. And this is the moment. If you want to honor yourself, you shall honor the teachings.

One day I was sleeping on an ordinary cot and my teacher came by my side. I just jumped up to greet him. He laughed and asked me to follow, so I followed him to his room. He said, "Is that a good yogi act to just jump to spring up like that?"

I said, "No my sir. It is not right. I know. But, I was caught in such a situation between a rock and a hard place when I saw you. I wanted to be respectful and I just got up."

"Is there any other reason?"

"No. I just wanted to greet you."

"You woke up."

"That's true."

---

[8] The Age of Aquarius is the age of experience. It is the age humanity is currently moving into. We are leaving behind the Age of Pisces, which is the age of belief.
[9] Projection: the way you act, move and deliver in time and space.

"You felt it?"

"That's true."

"And you jumped up?"

"That's true."

He said, "You have earned self-control. Now you can go."

I came back and one friend of mine asked me, "What did he say?"

"He told me I have earned self-control."

"What? Jumping up is self-control? Then, let's all jump."

And we said, "Okay, let's all jump."

Then some other students came and we started jumping. Just like kids do crazy things. We were in that kind of a mood. So we were jumping and our teacher came up and said, "Well, jumping does not give people self-control, monkeys."

And they said, "No, no, sir. He went and he jumped and you said, 'You have got self-control.' Well, sir, we started jumping, too."

He said, "No. His was a conscious jump. You are jumping just to jump. That is the difference between the two jumps. Now you can jump if you want—it's good exercise. Keep on jumping. But know that it has a purpose."

A life that does not have purpose and projection is a useless life. It is fortunate that everybody knows the purpose of life. The purpose of life is to be beautiful, to be bountiful, to be blissful, to be graceful and grateful. What a wonderful English word—grateful. If one is great and full, one is God. And whenever smallness faces you, you should be great. And full. Full of that greatness.

Some of you might be thinking, "What should we do? Why do we have to do it? Why are we here? Why are we not somewhere else?" Judge not my friends, or you shall be judged. Do not isolate yourself or you will be desolate. Don't go away or you will be gone. Self-discipline is to honor oneself, to honor the ideal of oneself.

It is very difficult for western civilization to understand the word, "surrender." When you surrender, you do not become weak or a slave. You exalt yourself. The touch of the master is not a fantasy. The touch of the Master is God's will. That man may be weaker, uglier and judgmental in your eyes, but if in the ecstacy of his consciousness if he blesses thee, thou shall always dwell in Thee. These are the ways of life. Dormant spirituality can be awakened by the touch of such a one.

Who are you in the progression of life? The future. And that's a fact. A teacher doesn't have anything. A teacher has no relatives. A teacher has no wealth, no riches. A teacher has a very simple touch—a very wishful touch. Because a teacher has to live with the student forever. Nanak was a teacher. He lives even today through his students. Not good. Not bad. Not great. Not small. It's a cosmology of the heavens in which those stars shine and they carry the words of Nanak, they carry the words of Jesus, they carry the words of Moses. Whether

Moses was great or small, Jesus was right or wrong, Nanak was fat or thin—forget all that. It is not the person, it is the person's words that have been infused, have been told and have brought faith and courage.

ਅਵਲਿ ਅਲਹ ਨੂਰੁ ਉਪਾਇਆ ਕੁਦਰਤਿ ਕੇ ਸਭ ਬੰਦੇ ॥
ਏਕ ਨੂਰ ਤੇ ਸਭੁ ਜਗੁ ਉਪਜਿਆ ਕਉਨ ਭਲੇ ਕੋ ਮੰਦੇ ॥੧॥

Aval alah noor upaa-i-aa kudrat kay sabh banday.
Ayk noor tay sabh jag upji-aa ka-un bhalay ko manday. ||1||

First is God and from His light everybody is born.
How can you say this is good and this is bad?

— Kabir ji, Siri *Guru Granth Sahib*, page 1349, line 19, as translated by Yogi Bhajan

When it came to Nanak, all he said was, "You are one God and one God's creation." When some fanatics got to him, he said, *Ram jap, Ram jap, hirdai Ram basat hai.* Chant *Ram*. Ram means "Maker of the sun and the moon" and it lives in the heart. So everywhere the faculty and the quality and the projection is in that Oneness. It's not in duality.

Maya has a duality. "I am myself. I am for myself. I am for my children. This is my home. This is my state. This is my country. This is my nationality." But if you really want to understand, there is nothing that you have. The body is a tool. The ribcage is a prison. It's a cage for the soul. If your soul is not happy in the ribcage, in your chest, you have not understood your very existence. If your breath is not easy, you have not respected life. If you see a very ugly, dirty, undesirable person and you have not reached out to comfort that soul and its existence, you have not learned anything. You talk of passionate love. You talk of possessions. You talk of everything. In reality, you have no possessions. Whatever you have is not yours. Your very body, its features, its shape, its faculty are not yours. Some people are shortsighted. Some are long sighted. Some have thick noses. Some have small noses. Some are tall. You have no control over it.

All right, you don't believe in God. I don't want to force you. But something else controls all. And when something else controls all, then let *all* be understood. Don't become an isolated individual. All is all. Even in small S-M-A-L-L, all is. All is contained in small.

Once, Milarepa[10] was walking and his teacher started abusing him. He took a stick and started beating him. Milarepa didn't know what he had done. He didn't understand it. First he tried to run. Then he stopped and put his hands down, and started getting beaten. He received the abuse. The teacher said, "Is that enough?"

Milarepa asked, "What enough?"

The teacher said, "I have beaten you so much."

"My lord, what do you mean by enough?"

"I have beaten you so much and I have abused you so much. Is it enough?"

---

[8] Jetsun Milarepa was a yogi and Buddhist saint from Tibet. He lived from 1052-1135.

"You know better than I."

"What do I know?"

Milarepa said, "There is that boulder, that huge stone, which by calamity was going to come and crush me. It would have rushed over me and crushed my bones. But it is still hanging there. It stopped moving because you started beating me and abusing me. And if that's enough, fine with me."

Then Milarepa ran and picked up his teacher and they rolled down the hill. That huge boulder gave way, following them as it rolled and rolled thundering on the earth. When they got to the bottom of the hill he asked his teacher.

"My lord, is that enough?"

Time and its actions or reactions, sequence and consequences can be diverted, not stopped. Everything can be diverted to safety by graceful action. That is *dharma*. All the tragedies that are supposed to hit you can be avoided and made minimal.

But when we see the sequence and we see the consequences, we freak out. We are not grateful. We do not understand that good has no limit. The same with bad. For thousands of years we have been taught that everything is ours, everything is our action, everything is under our control. This is my property. This is my son. This is my daughter. This is my religion. This is my guru. This is my God.

But isn't it the same God? Isn't it the same guru? Isn't it the same temple? Isn't it the same worship? You can sit on your heels or you can stand up on one leg. Whatever you do, isn't the One all there is? We have never understood the message of Nanak. "In One," he said. Nobody has understood the words *"Ek Ong Kaar." Ek Ong Kaar* doesn't need anything but the recognition that I am one with every one. In every one is *Ek Ong Kaar*. That is how the Shabad Guru[11] started, with that one phrase—*Ek Ong Kaar*. People are so shy to understand it—to be it.

When you sweat and hassle, you will never get royalty. You will not get bounty. It's not that you don't deserve bounty or that you don't deserve prosperity, but you are a thief. You are stealing a part of you from the One. Therefore you will get only a part. You will not get the whole.

You make fences. All right. You're controlling yourself, "I am me. I am for myself." Thank you very much. But when prosperity comes, it will find all the hurdles you, yourself, have created. You are not for all. You are not for, *Sarbat da bala*—goodwill for humanity.

> *Your prosperity is what your manners are. Your power is how your mind is. Your strength is what your mutuality is. Your business is what your negotiation is. Your grace is what your character is.*

---

[11] **Shabad Guru** is the practice of meditating upon the words of enlightened masters as a way to awaken one's spirit. The **Shabad Guru** is embodied in the **Siri Guru Granth Sahib**, a compilation of 1430 pages of sacred teaching songs written by the Sikh masters and other masters who were their contemporaries.

You are not unique and open to all winds. That was the beauty of the tall ships. The trade winds would blow. They could change their direction, grab the wind and sail the ship. Had those winds not existed, they never would have sailed.

This life of yours is meant to be a life of all within you and all existing in you. God is omnipresent and omnipotent. So are you. When you say, "I am not this. I am not that. I am not here. I am not there," who are you talking to? Every lie you have ever spoken has been understood later by another man. Why start a lie that has to be understood later? Why start a sequence for which you are not willing to face the consequences? You have a life. You have a responsibility. If honor has been bestowed on you, carry that honor and honor everybody. That honor is no good that cannot honor others. That grace is no good that cannot shower grace. That power is no good that cannot uplift others. That knowledge is no good that cannot comfort and give the heavens to others.

You are a human. It is your *dharma* to show the light and the path to all. It is your day. It has dawned for you. It is your gift. You must carry your *dharma*, your duty. Let your memory ever be that you will uplift everything. What is wrong with being social? What's wrong with meeting others? Why do you act like baboons jumping all the time? Why do you talk about miseries all the time? All this karma adds up.

Your prosperity is what your manners are. Your power is how your mind is. Your strength is what your mutuality is. Your business is what your negotiation is. Your grace is what your character is. My friends, everything is in you. You can protect yourself, or the One who made you can protect you. Never lose your innocence, and the Heavenly Father and Mother Nature shall always protect you. As it was in the beginning when you were children, so shall it be now. And you shall be guarded until the end.

There are two ways to live life. Either you will be guarded or you will be goaded by time and space and be miserable. You may have everything, but you will have no joy. Where God is not indulged in, there is no amount of satisfaction. Rich and poor is maya. Healthy and sick is maya. There may be an unhealthy body, but a very healthy mind and a very enlightened spirit. Pay reverence to the co-existence of the entire humanity. And acknowledge in an affirmation that you are God. Within existence, the *atma* (the soul) and Paramatma (the Great Soul) are not two—they are not different. *Mahakal* and *Akal* have no *kaal* to face[12]. In this grace, you must exist forever. Opportunities and callings will come and knock at your door. There is a mastermind that will give your mind the indication. Once grace is bestowed upon you, never let it go. Put yourself into it. Learning to dwell in God is learning to dwell in your grace.

---

[12] *Mahakal*: Cosmic Time. *Akal*: Timelessness. *Kaal*: Regular time.

Learning to dwell in God
is learning to dwell in
your grace.

Chapter Four

The Breath of Life
is a Gift to Share

There is a simple line:

ਬਿਨੁ ਭਾਗਾ ਸਤਸੰਗੁ ਨ ਲਭੈ ਬਿਨੁ ਸੰਗਤਿ ਮੈਲੁ ਭਰੀਜੈ ਜੀਉ ॥੩॥

Bin bhaagaa satsang na labhai bin sangat mail bhareejai jee-o. ||3||

Without gathering together in the company of that spirituality in which we get rid of
duality and sit in Oneness under the guidance of Guru and God in our own being;
without this, our behavior becomes dirty.

— Guru Ram Das, *Siri Guru Granth Sahib*,
Page 95, Line 10, as translated by Yogi Bhajan

What dirt are we talking about? We become shortsighted. What is longsighted?
Longsighted is that intuitive self in which a person has personal confidence. With the sense
of *Ang Sang Wahe Guru*[13,] you keep going. It's not that one doesn't look for opportunities

---

[13] *Ang Sang Wahe Guru:* my every molecule vibrates to the greatness of that wisdom that takes me from darkness to light.

and tragedies at the same time. This world is a mirage. And in this mirage many people, temporarily or permanently, have fallen apart. It's a mirage and it's a gorge, too. Once you slip, it's bottomless—it's endless.

Technically speaking, life is very positive when it is content. Life doesn't come to you because you are very wise. Life comes to you when you are very content, when you are sober and when you are trustworthy. Then people will like you. They will open up their hearts to you and give you opportunities. Thus life explains itself.

But unfortunately, some people have such a short circuit in the realm of their own consciousness that they do not enjoy their life and the light of their own life.

Corruption is in our genes. Though without the breath of life, the genetic corruption is useless. It means death. Still, with our genetic corruption we think we are living, but it is not true. The breath is living in us. This body is a structure in which the breath of life lives. Why does it live? Because it has a karma. It has come here at a certain longitude and latitude. It has collected two parents to do it. It is born when the environments are useful and then it goes. Whatever you are getting in life normally is already predestined—because your birth is predestined, your parents are predestined, your relatives are predestined, and your environments are predestined. Therefore, what you earn here in goodwill, compassion, grace and kindness is through discipline.

If you are a Muslim and you call everybody who is not a Muslim an infidel, that is not *dharma*. That is not religion. If you are a Christian and you don't relate to anybody who is not Christian, that is not *dharma*. If you are a Jew and you say, "I am the chosen one and everybody else is nothing," that is not *dharma*. Whenever you reach a saturated point, you are a dead idiot because your flexibility is gone.

When your physical flexibility is gone, you are very sick and when your mental flexibility is gone, you are very, very sick. It doesn't give you anything. There is nothing, no sin you can commit and there is no nice graceful thing you can do. The only question is how flexible you are.

Ultimately, today, tomorrow or the next day, this body will become stiff. There is no way around it. It will consume itself because the breath of life will not be consumed.

That's why *pranayam*[14] is the way of life. We're not asking that everybody should do yoga. Oh, it is an eastern thing. Oh, it is a western thing. What does that mean? Eastern and Western thing? My east is New York. My west is Hawaii. What is east and west? We have made phrases to demarcate ourselves and separate ourselves from life. This is Chinese. This is Japanese. This is American. This is Canadian. We have marked the world by boundaries and have divided people by signs, symptoms and language. It is amazing. Our life is amazing. We live on one Earth and one universe and yet we are not universal. We are not. And the worst thing that has happened to us is our spirituality. Spirituality has become about power.

Not to understand compassion is not to understand God. God is an impulse of expansion and man is a compassionately understanding expansion. However much you don't understand, that much you contract. And if you are contracted, then what is the use of life? Do you know each other? No. You work hard your whole life, and never know each other. That's the first law to remember.

---

[14] *Pranayam* – yogic breathing practices.

The only thing you will know, when you are compassionate and as vast as the ocean, is that everybody else is like a little boat on it. Everybody is a part of you. If you do not understand that everybody is a part of you then you do not understand who you are.

You know, on every corner of the road there is a synagogue, there is a temple, there is a church, there are swamis and yogis. There are a lot of people and a lot of teachings. The libraries are full. There are so many organizations, it is unbelievable. But nobody is there to tell you that you are an idiot. They won't. But the problem is not that they don't want to say that you are an idiot. The problem is that if they say you are an idiot then you will say, "Okay, make me a non-idiot." That is where they get stuck.

From the pulpit, in the name of Christ, there are so many lectures you can't believe it. But he practiced fasting. Do they? Have they practiced anything from his life that is still living? Anything? No. It's not possible.

We have come to go. Have we prepared ourselves for going? We are always ready to come. Coming is important and going is not. Yet, go we must. Know we must. And the most important thing is we must show that we are ready to go. If you understand that, you will never fight with anybody, you will never hate anybody and you will never squeeze anybody. It will be very difficult then for you to separate yourself from the universe at large.

I have seen people in my life who are very, very fanatically religious and then all of a sudden they break. And then there is nothing. Because when they were religious they were very, very squeezed into themselves. They were not vast. Religion is a reality that is very vast. You identify yourself with religion. That doesn't mean you are special, that means you are general. That means you will hug those who do not deserve to be helped. You misunderstand the meaning of religion. Religion is your own reality. Deep in you, there is a reality.

You may see things happening around you that you don't like. You can politely protest. When I came to the United States I had a chance to meet with many great people and I used to laugh. I would say, "You are already great, what do you want out of me?" But they had a different greatness. They had greatness of wealth. They had greatness of beauty. They had power. They were this and that. They were everything but themselves. And I understood when I left Hollywood that being worshipped by these people is useless, because they have a habit. They have an emptiness. They are hungry for spiritual growth but they don't want to work for their spirit. They can't.

I once asked a lady, "Do you know how much wealth you have got?"

She said, "I can call my head accountant."

"You do not know how wealthy you are?"

"No, I have never bothered. I don't know how wealthy I am. All I know is when I want to spend money, I get it."

"Do you know how many dresses you have got?"

"Well, there is a switch. If you start that, there is a laundry roller."

Around that whole house there was a ten-foot wide laundry roller on which her dresses were hanging. She would put a number into a computer and press the button and that dress would come, so she could take it out.

I counted. The lady had 17 fur coats, all different colors.

I asked her, "Do you ever wear them?"

"Sometimes. Why are you asking me these questions?"

"Sit down. You will fall over when I explain it to you."

"I'd like to know why you are asking these questions."

I said, "You do not even know who you are—that is a separate question. But you do not know how much you have. If you do not know how much you have on this Earth, then you will not know what you have hereafter. Is there something for over there? One day, you've got to go. Do you have something?"

"Where am I going? I am not going anywhere."

"You are going one day. You will go."

"Okay, explain it to me. I'll agree if you explain it to me."

I said, "How many poor people have you fed? How many poor people have you clothed? Forget about humans. How many birds have you fed? How many trees have you planted? How many times have you fasted?"

"Is it necessary to fast?"

"Yes. To give the body a break once in a while, you should fast and not eat."

"Oh that is fasting?"

I said, "Yes." She didn't know the meaning of fasting. Is that life?

She asked, "Why should we fast?"

"It gives us stamina. It gives us control over our hunger. That's why we fast. Self-control is the way of life. Sharing your own life with yourself is the way of life."

Closing your eyes and meditating is self-control, trying to calm yourself down. You can fight with your mind better. These are simple things that people don't understand.

It's very funny. Those who have to give have to act like God. But they don't give. And when you cannot give, then you possess. And when you posses, you are very scared. When you are scared, then you are very insecure. And when you are insecure and you feel horrible, terrible and miserable, then life has pain in it.

ਘਰਿ ਤ ਤੇਰੈ ਸਭੁ ਕਿਛੁ ਹੈ ਜਿਸੁ ਦੇਹਿ ਸੁ ਪਾਵਏ ॥

Ghar ta tayrai sabh kicch hai jis day-eh so paava-ay.

God, you have everything in you. In your home.
You give to whom you want to give.

— Guru Amar Das[15], *Anand Sahib*, Pauree 3,
as translated by Yogi Bhajan

---

[15] Guru Amar Das, Third Guru or Master in the Sikh Tradition. He lived from 1479-1574.

God is willing to give but are we willing to receive? Giving is a rational flow; When God gives, we give, too. Out of His will, we give. Out of our will, we control.

Dasvandh is the practice of tithing in which we give 10% out of the 100% of everything that God has given to us. Is there any place where you can keep 90% and still feel miserable?

Dasvandh is when you give 10% out of what you have been given as seed money. And you get to keep 90%. But still we don't understand. You forget to give your 10%.

Our rational living is very simple. The breath of life on which we live is given by God. Our life is actually a testimony to the fact somebody makes us live. We don't understand that. We just understand that we live. Isn't it surprising that the breath of life is given to us and there are no guarantees?

ਹਮ ਆਦਮੀ ਹਾਂ ਇਕ ਦਮੀ ਮੁਹਲਤਿ ਮੁਹਤੁ ਨ ਜਾਣਾ ॥

Ham aadmee haan ik damee muhlat muhat na jaanaa.

We are human beings of the briefest moment;
we do not know the appointed time of our departure.

— Guru Nanak, *Siri Guru Granth Sahib*,
Page 660, Line 11

I am just a one-breath man. Breath comes and then it goes. That's all it is. And when it cannot come, it cannot go. We create environments that have so much pressure, weight, walls, values, virtues, status—all according to our conception. And then we suffer. Why do we suffer? Actually, the fact is that we want to suffer. If we are relaxed we will never suffer.

I once knew a very beautiful psychiatrist. He was my student when I taught at UCLA, and he was upset all the time. He was upset with his car. He was upset with his home. He was upset with his wife. He was upset with the children.

I asked him about it. He said, "It's my habit."

I said, "You are reaching the end of your life. Your blood pressure is high. You sometimes even lose consciousness and still you are upset?

"I don't know how to stop it."

"Well, lie down someplace for ten, fifteen minutes and close your eyes and breathe long and deep."

He got totally cured. Totally. And he told me, "That was the easiest medicine I ever had."

I said, "It is always there."

When you do not know what to do, just take a long, deep breath because your life is based on the breath. The shorter the breath, the worse off you are. The longer the breath, the better you are.

Dasvandh

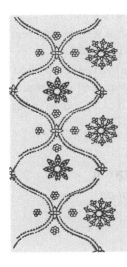

Editor's Note: When the Siri Singh Sahib, Yogi Bhajan, talked about the practice of Dasvandh, he often addressed two aspects of it. On the one hand, he talked about the blessings that come from consciously giving back to your spiritual source—however you define it. The other point was specifically addressed to the Sikh community, explaining that Dasvandh was a time-honored way for the community to build itself and its future. Here, we have included some passages from both perspectives relating to Dasvandh—the general benefits of tithing, and the overall strength of a community consciously giving to its own future.

Dasvandh is a personal dictate. It is not a command. It cannot be discussed. I cannot share anything with you about it. It's a self-dictate. *Dasvandh* is a self-dictate, not a command.

When you give, you get. Without *Dasvandh*, you give nothing. Because *Dasvandh* is the one time you give in the name of the Creator, Almighty God, and you get back many times for it. So giving is an art of living. It is the Age of Experience. Therefore, it becomes blindingly essential for us to give. I know it is hard. But it is hard to take and live with it. Those who balance themselves by giving *Dasvandh* have the blessing of God and Guru.

Any offering given in the name of God or any offering given in the self-exertion of the unknown multiplies faster than an offering in time and space. It is a mental attribution and it is a physical contribution. The attribution and the contribution blend together by the individual's act.

Why do you give? Nobody asks you to give. Why do you want to give? You don't want to give. So why do you give? Because you are giving it. There is no rational reason.

Something moves this earth. Something makes time and space. So we should give a little bit to that. How much? One tenth. Why one tenth? *Dasvandh* means one tenth. One is the Creator. Zero is infinity. So the Creator unto Infinity makes one tenth. One over one tenth. These things are not unknown mysteries. These are known masteries. One tenth of your wealth. Not that somebody wants your one tenth. To whom do you give? You give it to yourself because everything you give returns to you ten-fold.

Similarly, giving two and a half hours of your time to the unknown is also *Dasvandh*. Time and space—there are these two things. We give in the form of money for space. We give in the form of meditation, chanting, kirtan, and all those activities in the form of time. When you blend time and space with the unknown you become the beloved of the unknown.

Sikh Dharma has a very good practice, though sometimes you are unable to enjoy it. It makes you you. It gives you your higher You. All other activities give you the satisfaction of a performance. But the activities in Sikh Dharma give you the satisfaction of you. That's why in Guru Nanak's house, ritual has no place. Contribute one tenth of you to you. Contribute one tenth of you to your higher being. Give yourself a chance.

For the Khalsa

Dasvandh is the old way to tie in one tenth of your earnings to the house of the Guru so things can run—and run at your own accord and by your own will. All of you as a body of the Khalsa should try to take the burden.

You don't give *Dasvandh*. You say, "*Dasvandh* for what?" I'll tell you for what. So that you can die somewhere gracefully. I'm not saying that you should give all your money. Actually *Dasvandh* belongs to the Guru. It doesn't belong to you. That money belongs to the Guru and that money is for the future. That money is for YOUR future, for your children's future, for your grandchildren's future.

We have to have a school. We have to have a home and things for old people. We have to have things for children and young people. We have to have so many things. And they have to come from the Guru's money, not your money.

If everybody gives one tenth and it's all done for your coming generations to learn, to grow and to be—is there any better investment than that?

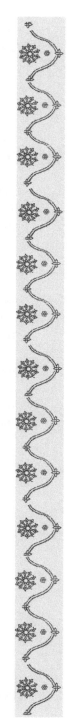

Recently there was a problem. There was a girl who was in love and things were not happening right. You know what I mean? Love does that. There's a lot of passion, a lot of feelings, a lot of thinking. These are the signs of lovers. They don't eat. They are just negative about everything. They philosophize about everything. They talk very high and they do not even know where the ground is. "Oh, I see him, I see him, I see him …" It goes on like that.

One day she called and she said, "I am in too much pain. Things are not happening right." I said, "Count your breaths per minute."

She was breathing thirty-five breaths per minute. Thirty-five! Normal breathing is fifteen and a well-balanced person breathes ten times a minute. If you are really a practitioner and you want to be prosperous then you have to breathe within seven and nine breaths a minute. Fewer than that—you are a yogi. If you want things done for you and you don't want to have to do anything, then you must breathe from one to five or six breaths per minute. If you can practice this then you can attract the universe to you. It is not a secret. It's a simple thing. The longer and deeper the breath is, the more your psyche attracts everything for you, and that's a way to prosperity.

There are some people who are perpetually a failure. Everything fails. This thing doesn't work, that thing can't. If you tell them to practice ten breaths a minute, and meet them after two or three years, they will be so prosperous and so beautiful. Because the sense of their communication changes. There is fear in your voice. If you can eliminate that fear, you can surely be prosperous. If you are wealthy you will enjoy wealth. Because the living psyche is part of you and that decides everything.

I know one person who is a counselor. You know what he does? He puts a person in a chair and tells him to vibrate the lips like this, "burrrrrrrrrrrr." After half an hour, the person gets tired of it, but the person is so relaxed. When you hate somebody you do this, burrrrrrrrrrrr. He makes people do this and nothing else, and they get so relaxed and so tired that sometimes they fall asleep. Their lives change.

ਸੈਲ ਪਥਰ ਮਹਿ ਜੰਤ ਉਪਾਏ ਤਾ ਕਾ ਰਿਜਕੁ ਆਗੈ ਕਰਿ ਧਰਿਆ ॥

Sail pat'har meh jant upaa-ay taa kaa rijak aagai kar dhari-aa.

For even those creatures who were made to be born in the stones,
God has provided their food and meals.

— Guru Arjan, *Rehiraas Sahib*,
as translated by Yogi Bhajan

I asked him, "But aren't you supposed to counsel them?"

He said, "Counsel with what? They are burrrrrrrrrrrr their whole life, so I make them do it openly and clearly so that they can get tired of it. The moment they get tired, they sleep. And when they get up they are new people. Slowly and gradually they are building their sense of self."

You are constantly fighting. When you sit, you fight. When you eat, you fight. You fight with everything. And do you think by yelling and screaming, by raising your voice and attacking something that you are going to get something? No. You should never alert the psyche of another person no matter what. Never ever challenge the psyche of another person. If the frequency of the other person is more than two points, God is going to get you forever. There is no need for it.

If God made you to be then, "To be to be." You want to know something? If somebody is very rude and crude with you, just laugh. See how miserable the other person feels and enjoy it. Because that anger, that projection and that rejection of that self will all come out in one big blast. And if you laugh a little more, then they will say, "Shut up. What are you doing? You are mocking me. Bah-bah-bah." And then the dog will come out, barking.

Are we human or dogs? Our intelligence and our sophistication are the keys to our living. Sometimes I wonder if we have learned to give. There is something called the reverse cycle. When you have to give and you don't give, the cycle reverses on you. Then it takes away all that you have. It's a very magnetic principle to understand. There is nothing more difficult than understanding it. Nanak said,

ਦੇਦਾ ਦੇ ਲੈਦੇ ਥਕਿ ਪਾਹਿ ॥
ਜੁਗਾ ਜੁਗੰਤਰਿ ਖਾਹੀ ਖਾਹਿ ॥

Daydaa day laiday thak paahi.
Jugaa jugantar khaahee khaahi.

The One who gives, gives. Those who take get tired. And that's the misery of life.

— Guru Nanak, *Japji Sahib*, Pauree 3, as translated by Yogi Bhajan

ਹੁਕਮੀ ਹੁਕਮੁ ਚਲਾਏ ਰਾਹੁ ॥
ਨਾਨਕ ਵਿਗਸੈ ਵੇਪਰਵਾਹੁ ॥੩॥

Hukmee hukam chalaa-ay raahu.
Naanak vigsai vayparvaahu. ||3||

Here is the problem. He gives and He commands. And that command is that which He gives. What a subtle thing to understand. What a simple thing to understand.

— Guru Nanak, *Japji Sahib*, Pauree 3,
as translated by Yogi Bhajan

Once a *sadhu* was going around and he came upon a man who was sitting and was very sad. The *sadhu* stopped and he said, "Baba, I am not supposed to ask this, but you seem to be very sad."

"Why not ask? I am very sad."

The *sadhu* said, "What are you doing sitting here?"

"Please don't ask. This is my lonely hour."

"What you are lonely about?"

"I have fourteen wives and twenty-four children and I have four palaces in this town. You see those big buildings? Do you see that?"

"Yes, I see it."

"Out of the window of that one building, I slip away. I am wearing ordinary clothes so nobody recognizes me. And I come here and I lament and lament and lament and cry."

"Why? Why you are crying? You have so much."

"That much is that much trouble. I have no contentment. I have no comfort."

"Are you for real? Look, hundreds and thousands of people do not have that much."

"That's what I come here to think about. I can give it to those hundreds and thousands of people who don't have it. I want to get rid of that torture and teasing; those problems and worries. That's not life."

The *sahdu* looked at him and said, "It looks like you have never eaten."

"No, I can't digest any food."

"How do you live?"

"I live on nothing."

The *sadhu* said, "Come here. Sit here. I feel very comfortable. Right now I am very comfortable."

So the *sadhu* took off his shawl, gave it to the man, put it around him and said, "Okay, if you have to sit here, at least you should not sit in this pose."

The moment the *sadhu* put the shawl around the man there was peace and tranquility. His life became very bubbly. The man felt very good. After a while he said, "Wait a minute, that man only had one shawl on his body and he gave it to me and then he left. In my home, there are a closet full of shawls. That's no good."

So the man ran around trying to find that *sadhu* but he couldn't. He wandered and wandered and wandered, but he couldn't find him. Finally, he came to a place under some trees and he saw the same *sadhu* sitting very tranquilly, peacefully enjoying his time. The man went up to him and he said, "Baba you must be feeling cold."

The *sadhu* laughed and said, "I am not you. I am very warm. You are cold."

"Your shawl has changed my life."

"Because the shawl has that vibration, those feelings I shared with you. You can have it."

Then the man asked the *sadhu* to come along with him to his house. At first, the *sadhu* was hesitant, but then he agreed. He came. When he came to the house, the man ordered things around and wanted to get the servants. The *sadhu* laughed so hard.

The man asked, "Baba, why are you laughing?"

The *sadhu* said, "Look, since I have entered this house, you are ordering everybody around. How many servants do you have?"

"Three hundred."

"Well, how good can life be? Three hundred people for one meal? This is all I want to eat."

And the *sadhu* took some chapatti[16], put some dal[17] on it, rolled it up and started eating. This man was looking at the gold plates and gold cups, all adorned with precious stones.

---

[16] Indian flat bread
[17] Indian lentils

But the *sadhu* said, "Those who have become the closest to Infinity live by the simplest of means. You have created complications. All this paraphernalia that you have created is to show your riches. But true riches are in your feeling of relaxation and contentment when you feel God is with you and God feels you are with Him."

The *sadhu* continued, "That's the relationship. Let's both eat."

And that was the first day the man digested his food. He ate and he felt content.

So that's what it is all about. What we have, what we feel, what we think, what we condemn, what we accept, what we reject, what we ask. Do we really feel it is the same inflow of infinity into our finite that is creative? That's what Nanak said. In that one line, he said,

ਅਨੰਦੁ ਭਇਆ ਮੇਰੀ ਮਾਏ ਸਤਿਗੁਰੂ ਮੈ ਪਾਇਆ ॥

Anand bha-i-aa mayree maa-ay satguroo mai paa-i-aa.

I am in ecstasy, O my mother, for I have found my True Guru.
— Guru Amar Das, *Anand Sahib*, Pauree 1

My bliss has come from the true Guru. Oh my Creative Mother, my basic intelligence, my sense of existence; I have found it from the true Guru. And that's why I am in bliss.

ਸਤਿਗੁਰੁ ਤ ਪਾਇਆ ਸਹਜ ਸੇਤੀ ਮਨਿ ਵਜੀਆ ਵਾਧਾਈਆ ॥

Satgur ta paa-i-aa sahj saytee man vajee-aa vaadhaa-ee-aa.

I have found the True Guru, with intuitive ease, and my mind vibrates with the music.
I have found it in a very novel and very humble way. And my mind is rejoicing.

— Guru Amar Das, *Anand Sahib,* Pauree 1, as translated by Yogi Bhajan

Sometime we just read these statements because Nanak spoke them. They are with us but we do not ponder over them. We do not walk along our route with them, we take them as routine. That's the difference.

We must understand our life is for expansion and it will keep expanding, until death, whether we use it or not. If we use our life it will expand beautifully. It will benefit us beautifully. It will make us comfortable beautifully. But you can't stop expansion. You were born like this, and you keep on growing.

Old age without wisdom, youth without success and childhood without smiles are worthless. Children must smile, youth must succeed and old age must be wise. These are the criteria upon which a person has to grow religiously. Self-expansion cannot stop. It keeps on growing.

> Who is your first enemy
> and your first friend?
>
> Your own mind.

Without meditation, the mind cannot be used. It becomes crooked. It has no boundaries. Who is your first enemy and first friend? Your own mind. Your mind works in your sleep. It works when you're awake. It works all the time. And when you don't meditate, the mind has no direction. It is a car that can hit any pole.

Sometimes, you use certain words. "Don't disturb me."

Somebody wants to talk to you and you say, "Don't disturb me. I am not in a good mood." I am just telling you your idiocy. "I am not in a good mood." How rude it is that you are not in good mood. You are a human being. If somebody comes to talk to you, how bad is it? You are supposed to see, meet head-on and receive that person. Learn to receive the psyche of another human being. Don't see the body; see the projection of the energy. If you cannot see God in all, you cannot see God at all. You can only see God in all if you know you have God in you. God meets the God. Devil doesn't meet the God.

Learn that you are beautiful if you don't speak. And when you speak, you must speak wisely. For that you need courage, self-confidence and sweetness. In the beginning there was the word. The word was with God and the word was God. Therefore every word you speak affects each one of us.

I wonder whether you know the beauties of the kriyas[18] that you have been given. They are great—I worked at the cost of my health to share them. For twenty-five years, I never sat still, never had a regular life. I ran from one place to another, from one congregation to another and we built up a knowledgeable community. I have failed in that I have not built up a practicing community. I tried my best. But you know more than you think you know. You simply have to digest it now.

My hope is that all of you will study every line of *Siri Guru Granth*[19] and will understand it and prepare yourself for the Age of Aquarius so you can make people understand the guidance of the way. Through that guidance you will find life happy and blissful. Then you will stop fighting and start receiving. Your joy lies in that reception and you will become beautiful, bountiful and blissful. That's life.

If you do not spread this knowledge and do not serve people, you will be guilty. It is not a matter of ego. It is not a matter of being recognized. The benefits of these practices will be recognized. These days yoga is very popular, it's a trend. And people have done everything. They have taken Prozac. They have taken everything. It didn't work. They have counseling, psychology, psychiatry. What is not available? But what is there which is not for the self.

---

[18] *Kriyas*: reference to Kundalini Yoga meditations and sets of exercises that create specific effects in the body, mind and spirit.
[19] *Siri Guru Granth Sahib*: form of the **Shabad Guru**. The collected writings of the Sikh Masters and other saints that, when meditated upon, will awaken the consciousness of a person.

If the self starts working, it will take care of things. There is nothing more important than your self. There is no God but you. You have to change the frequency of your psyche and change the degree of your expansion in consciousness, and you have to understand the behavior of compassion. Then, whatever you want, a hundred times more than that will come. Don't live a beggar's life. "I want this, I want this, I want this." It doesn't work.

I can tell you from my experience. I have been dirt poor twice in my life and each time I was very rich to start with. You won't believe me. When I first lived in Toronto and I found there was vegetarian pizza, there was no greater joy. I could eat. Before that, if I went to any restaurant and said, "I want soup," they would say, "Oh no, sir. There is chicken stock in it."

And I would say, "Can you just make it for me without the chicken stock?"

And they would say, "No, this is our formula. We don't know anything else."

Don't be temperamentally poor and live like a beggar, "Give me this, give me that, God give me this."

God will give you what He has to give you. His computer never fails.

I came here with thirty-five dollars and I have left you with millions and millions of dollars. I have left it to you. I never brought anything and I am not going to take anything. Now you have to act responsibly. You have to act consciously. Multiply. Work to be more successful in the businesses. Make more money and help more people. Give them a space of peace and tranquility and grace. Let people trust you. That can only happen if you trust yourself. There is no worth if you don't have your own worth on this Earth. You know the power in you is the thought. Just feel fulfilled.

When you say, "God give me this, God give me that," all the time, then God says, "What is wrong with this guy?" God gives you everything. The problem is God doesn't have your ways. God is infinity and vastness. You are limited and small. It doesn't work.

What difference does it make if you are poor or you are rich if you have not tried to help somebody? If you do not develop the habit of being a forklift, you are worse than any tool on this planet. Be like a forklift. Lift somebody up—anybody—with no obligation. Put somebody on the trail. Let somebody move. Let things move. Feel happy about it. That is your happiness. You will be rewarded for it.

One day on television, I saw the most powerful thing that made me cry and laugh. An Afghani child was saying, "When the planes come, sometimes they drop food; sometimes they drop pamphlets; sometimes they bring bombs. We are very confused."

> *Be like a forklift.*
>
> *Lift somebody up—anybody—with no obligation.*
>
> *Put somebody on the trail.*
>
> *Let somebody move.*
>
> *Let things move.*
>
> *Feel happy about it.*
>
> *That is your happiness.*

We are not confused. We know we have to feed two and half million people. We know that we have to teach them that fanaticism doesn't work. We have to tell them that pain begets pain. This is a very strange war that you are fighting. It is not a war between countries. It is a war between the haves and the have-nots.[20]

The freedom we used to enjoy is gone, but still you have to live. You need sobriety and you need self-control now. You need consciousness and you need to live in peace and tranquility within yourself. Sometime there may be a one-mile long line that you need to stand in. You will need patience then.

Blessed are those who bless themselves. Gracious are those who understand their own grace. Kind are those who are kind to themselves and their being and their surroundings. And virtuous are those who feel the entire universe belongs to them and they belong to the universe by itself. May your Creator God guide you to these aspects of life so that you can live in peace and grace. Sat Nam.

---

[20] Yogi Bhajan was speaking at the start of the War on Terror when the USA invaded Afghanistan.

Everybody is a part of you.
If you do not understand
that everybody is a part
of you then you do not
understand who you are.

CHAPTER FIVE

TRUST GOD TO WORK FOR YOU

Today I will share with you some human secrets that will shock you. First, I will ask some questions.

How many of you want to be divine and experience ecstasy?

Almost everybody. Is that true? So if you want it, then why don't you get it? Every religion—no matter what you practice—means ecstasy, right? And you want to experience ecstasy—that's true. You should see through the Third Eye and see above all. That's a natural human desire. It's a privilege as a human and the way of prosperity. There's no denying it. But why don't you get it?

It is not a discipline. That's the tragedy of it. God has nothing to do with it. There are two ways to live. One way is that you will hustle for prosperity. The other way is that prosperity will come to you. In one way, you would like to have a man and have sex and that is it. The other is that you will be worshipped and respected and the right partner will come.

Everything that is right shall come to you. And everything that just looks right shall go wrong for you. There are only two ways. You can check your own life without me saying one word and you will find that this is true. You will grab things in your hand and they will go sour. But when you have nothing to do with it, things will become sweet to you.

It's not trust. Trust is simply that you trust. When your mom says. "This is your father," you trust it whether you like it or not, so, who cares?

I'm not going into philosophy. Today, we are talking about very simple things. All that you have been taught is absolutely obsolete and wrong.

Nobody can accept anybody. Love is nothing but a playground. Do you know there is no such thing as love? A human is not competent to love. And when love happens, a human is not competent to stop it. You know that? When you love somebody, you can't stop it. But when you want to love somebody, you can do this whole rigmarole, and nothing happens. After a while, copper appears and the gold disappears. As long as your hot-blooded, sexual, marginal molecules are a little stronger in the blood, it's all "love." But when you are eighty years old, what you love most is not coughing. And not coughing is a great love.

Today is the first class in the Age of Aquarius. I am not teaching anything Piscean. We have started with Nanak and we are talking about the Age of Aquarius.

So, what can give you instant prosperity, divinity, reality and can wipe out your weaknesses? Should I give you the answer?

You believe in life. You believe in life. You believe that you have a father but you don't know for sure. There is a possibility that if you get a genetic test, you can find out whether he is your father. But the test is only 90% accurate so there is still a 10% doubt. You believe there is a mother. And you believe you live. You also believe you will get up tomorrow morning. You believe it. You do all this mischief with the hope that you will be living tomorrow. If you did not have this belief that you will live tomorrow, there are a million things you wouldn't do.

We believe. The fact is we believe. But we deny that we do a lot of things on belief. If I say I love you, it's a belief. Do you understand? Then you keep waiting. He said he loves me, but when? Where? Why? What? You process your beliefs all your life and that is the Piscean Age. That is the Piscean process—the fish going after the fish. You go after your thoughts. Your thoughts circulate. You believe.

But, even if you don't believe, God will believe in you. Your Creator will come through. Isn't it simple?

If you are a Sikh, every day you say: Nothing mine is in me. Everything is yours, Oh Lord.

But you don't believe that. Because you cannot let this man go. You believe you can make love. You believe you can have a relationship. You believe you will be rich. If you don't believe you will be rich, then you will be rich.

Read the poem I wrote in the book *The Man called Siri Singh Sahib*.

> *One day the day shall come*
> *When all the glory will be Thine.*
> *People will say, "It's yours."*
> *I shall deny, "Not mine."*

That poem was written when I was dirt poor and Mr. Nothing. People used to say that I prophesized, but I did not prophesize anything. There will be nine hundred sixty million people and there will be a sovereign nation and it's not for everybody.

Some of my benefactors in Hollywood were well-to-do. Once they said, "We can do this, this and this for you. Just come along."

I said, "No. I have to become what I have to become. I am just a postman. My only job is to take a bag of letters, deliver them and forget it. It's not my job to go, deliver the letter, open it, read it, translate it and make a person understand it. And then go to the next house. It would take a full day in only one place. That's not my job."

You can hate me. You can love me. But when you call on me, I will be there. That's what you have to believe. What do you have to believe? When there is a call, you are not there. God is. Because God is everywhere and in every way. So what is it that you have to believe?

ਖ਼ਾਲਸਾ ਮੇਰੋ ਰੂਪ ਹੈ ਖ਼ਾਸ ॥
ਖ਼ਾਲਸੇ ਮਹਿ ਹੌਂ ਕਰੋ ਨਿਵਾਸ ॥

Khaalsaa mero roop hai khaas
Khalsay meh ho karo nivaas.

Khalsa is my true form.
Within the Khalsa, I abide.

Guru Gobind Singh[21], the father of the Khalsa nation, said this in his own words.

He said it when he was alive—in a shape, in a form, in a person.

ਖ਼ਾਲਸਾ ਮੇਰੀ ਜਾਨ ਕੀ ਜਾਨ ॥

Khaalsaa mayree jaan kee jaan.

Khalsa is the breath of my life

— Guru Gobind Singh, from *Sarbloh Granth*

He made all these statements. He was alive. He could be felt. He could be heard.

So there are two theories of life. One is *Ik Gunn*, and the other is *Bahu Gunn*. This means God is one, He multiplies. And from multiples, He becomes One. The same applies to you.

You are here to watch and God is here to work. You want to do *seva* (service) for God? No, God will do *seva* for you. If I say that, the Sikhs will throw me out, but it's a fact.

God is there to be with you. God is there to create you and God is there creating you. God is there continuing the creativity. That's the quality of God. But you have to believe it.

You are all prosperous. Nature, *prakriti*, will serve you. When prakriti will serve you, you will have ecstasy. But you have to hold onto *purkha*. *Purkha* is that One. When you hold the One everything becomes shuniya—nothing. And all is zero then. So the zeros become ten, a hundred, a thousand, and it goes up to infinity.

---

[21] Guru Gobind Singh ji was the tenth10th master in the Sikh tradition. He lived from 1666-1708. During his lifetime, he initiated a discipline for the Sikhs to live as spiritual warriors. The Sikh practice of the spiritual warrior is known as the *Khalsa*.

You have to hold to one thought: God is creative, *Ek Ong Kaar*. Have you heard some foolish people chanting it like *Ek Om Kaar*? Have you heard that? They chant it and they want to correct you. Some person has the guts to say, "No Yogiji, it is *Ek Om Kaar*."

I tell them, "The universe is a sound. Do you know the difference? Get out of my sight. I don't want to spoil my ears."

I am not here to learn anything. I refuse to learn. Therefore, I refuse to teach. I just deliver. Don't you believe in delivering? Ask the woman who is pregnant. Tell her not to deliver and see what happens to her. What will happen to her? She will be dead.

When you have the spirit and you don't deliver, you will be the living dead.

A candle that does not burn is a dead candle. You want to be an attorney. You want to be a doctor. You want to be all these things. That has nothing to do with you being a human. Human. Hue-Mann. Hue means light. Mann means mental. If you do not light another mental light with your mental light, you are dead. And a dead person doesn't live prosperously.

I went to Los Angeles once and taught yoga classes. One student said, "I don't know. I am very much in love with this man, but I cannot reach him."

I said, "It's very good. You are in love with this man, right?"

"Don't say it. I know. I should try to reach Infinity."

"Yeah."

The third day, the guy came. He said, "I have ignored you."

You know, all these men have a very clever way of talking. They are the cleverest seducers on the planet. And they are hunters. Even 30 or 40 years after marriage, they are still hunters. You can't change their nature.

He will always say, "I love you." They do not know what love is because they do not have breasts. They cannot nurture.

Do we have breasts? They are flat. How can a flat guy nurture?

Their construction is defective. If they make love through their organ, downstairs between the legs, they can't say they are lovers. They are ejaculators. Do you understand what I am saying? You can't accept it. This is the Age of Aquarius. This language is different.

You only want to hear nice language. "God is merciful. God is very kind. I have seen the *Guru* with my own eyes. I was meditating. He came through me." Actually, meditation is for nothing other than for you to clear your shit. All thoughts in the subconscious that are negative, unfulfilled and wrong start floating to the surface. That's what meditation is. Meditation is nothing but cleaning a house with a vacuum. You create a vacuum for your thoughts. You clean and that's meditation. So that whole day you can be light, and polite. You can be nice, have endurance, have tolerance, and not freak out.

What is the best way you can win the world? Have you seen those books, act like this and win friends? What is that one principle that allows you to win the universe, the Creator, the creation, the contact, the consent, and everything? What is that practice? Stand before a mirror and smile. Keep on smiling. Even if you want to be dead, even if somebody is mad at you, just keep on smiling. See how fast he attacks you. You think a smile is not a power? It's the most powerful tool a human has.

Once I was teaching at Berkeley University and somebody started abusing me out of nowhere. The poor man was drunk and I kept smiling. I said, "Well, do more. Come on—more. A little more." He got so upset that he wanted to become physical. I said, "Come on and go ahead. Have fun."

A week later, I taught another class and he was in the class again. But this time he was a very good student. He acted nice. When I left the class, he came along with me and he said, "Well, I have one question."

I said, "What?"

"I was very negative and wanted to attack you that day. And I am sorry for that. But you were smiling."

"Yeah, I was."

"Why?"

"I was smiling because you don't know me. If perchance you had attacked me, God, I would have shredded you. I am a trained killer."

"Oh yeah, where did you learn?"

"Where your father studied. Aren't you the son of Corporal so and so from the sixth battalion?"

"How do you know?"

"I investigated. Your father beats you too much and you have anger. Therefore, you hate everybody who tells you what to do. I was teaching a class and I was telling you what to do so you became very angry with me."

"God, you know everything."

"No, I just know a part of it."

No human being has the desire to misbehave. So why do people misbehave? Because they are raised handicapped. They are raised handicapped and that's why they misbehave.

If somehow you can believe or trust that God has created you, then you understand Guru Nanak. That's what *Ek Ong Kaar* means. *Ek Ong Kaar*. This universe is created. This *prakriti* (nature) is created is by the One. And you are part of that One.

Have patience. Wait. Things will start happening. All prosperity is based on opportunities, correct? And all opportunities have to be cashed in, correct?

The opportunities will only be cashed in when the hand of the Creator is behind it. This is the biggest failure of a person—when they put their ego into something.

This life is he and her. That's why you chant. *Har, Har, Har.*[22]

Har is nurturing, creative. She has the breasts. You've got to learn those lessons. She nurtures you, nurses you, and enlarges you.

Scientifically, that's the faculty of the moon. That's why the moon wanes and waxes. That's how vegetables grow. That's how fruits grow. That's how the weather changes. That's how the oceans change. That's how the wind changes.

In the Age of Aquarius, what are you? When you will study everything, all books and all practices, and everything; and when God will appear before you and He says, "What do you want?" and you say, "Give me the ultimate knowledge." What will that be?

That *purkha* is the source of *prakriti*.

[22] *Har:* one of the mantras in Kundalini Yoga. It can be translated as the Essential Creativity of the Creator.

CHAPTER SIX

DEVELOP YOUR CROSS-REFERENCE

Today we are going to educate ourselves about "cross-reference." Do you know what cross-reference is? Two things you always know: you always know what is right and you always know why you are not doing what is right. When you know what is right and when you know that you cannot do what is right, at that time, if you have a cross-reference, you can hold yourself together. It is a temporary holding of the energy.

If we have not developed the cross-reference in ourselves, we will do wrong—knowingly and precisely. And we will pray that we can escape and not get caught. Mothers do it. Fathers do it. Doctors do it. Attorneys do it. Chief Executive Officers do it. This is a human failure.

In our personality, there is a very powerful computer. It's called consciousness. It's feeble. It's humble. It has a little voice. When you meet somebody, even at first sight, you know whether a person is trouble, or whether a person needs help, where the person has to go. And then you say, to heck with it. I have nothing to do with it.

Ninety percent of all our pain is because we have no cross-reference. There is nothing in us that we can look at as an experience of what is me and my soul, of what gives me the experience of Infinity. All I know is that this is planet earth. This is my home. This is my girl. This is my boy. This is my money. All I know is what is opaque. There is no gem quality. There is no cross-reference to see through like crystal.

A crystal is the most powerful thing. And what have we done? We have taken physical crystals and we hang them around our necks to satisfy us. Crystals are healing. If you become crystal, you are healed. And what is the crystal in you? The cross-reference. Right is right and wrong is wrong and you can see right or wrong. And your consciousness can tell you wrong is wrong and it cannot be right. When you have that strength, then—with cross-reference—you cross fire and say, "No." Do you know the joy of that no? Have you any idea? No. You don't. Ninety-nine point nine percent of people become victims because they don't have the capacity and authentic approach to say, "No."

Technologically, you have all the options of knowledge. If you say you don't have knowledge, you are lying to yourself.

ਬੀਜ ਮੰਤੁ ਸਰਬ ਕੋ ਗਿਆਨੁ

Beej mantar sarab ko gi-aan.

Within the sound of the seed lies all wisdom.

— Guru Arjan Dev ji, *Siri Guru Granth Sahib*, page 274, line 16

Your spermatozoa knows how to reach the egg. It may die reaching it, but it knows which way to run. It doesn't come back out. Do you know your body, your organs and your actions are all complete and perfect? Your molecules, your blood circulation, the beat of your heart and the movement of your lungs are so rhythmic. The only thing in you that is unrhythmic is you. Isn't it amazing that the entire body from top to bottom is totally rhythmic, and the only thing that is not rhythmic and harmonious is you? Because you clash with your ego, you are never you. Your ego is never yours. It never can be—because you do not know who you are. You don't know where to stop and you don't know where to start.

Your intellect gives you millions of thoughts. You start pursuing them blindly. When it becomes your desire, you cannot master your desire. And then you cannot master your life. Mastery is not a gimmick. Mastery is not spirituality. Mastery is life. That creates a legacy. When you don't have any option but to say "no" and if, at that time, you cannot exercise your "no," you have lost.

Work it out. Feel within yourself how many times you lose every day. When you have to say "yes" but you don't have the guts, strength, courage to say "yes." Why? Because your actions have no cross-reference. When you have no cross-reference, and you get caught, you don't admit it—out of guilt.

Admit it. Don't admit it to anybody else. Admit it to yourself. Do you know that people do not have a truthful relationship with themselves? Are you aware of that? Forget about whether somebody has a relationship with me or somebody has a relationship with you. People truly do not have a relationship with themselves. So what happens?

When you are young, you are pushed to a certain point of study or acknowledgment or work based on what the environments are. In middle age, you reach a certain stage where you have a certain status. And after that, there is the rest of your life. It starts at age forty-two. The sixth level of consciousness begins at forty-two.[23] You start living excuses. It's not that you are old. After forty, you don't become useless or old. These are all excuses.

If you are experienced, you are wise, and you have a cross-reference, and a cross wire and you can be you, it's such an enjoyable life. It's such a happy life that there is nothing to worry about.

What's your weight? What's your gravity? How much should somebody respect you and follow you and trust you? How long can you last? Everything is a business—friendships, relationships. You are a mixture of a lot of things. When there is heat every other material will burn, but gold will stay. Do you know that theory? And it will never change its gravity. The gold in you is your cross-reference, your capacity, your density, your beauty, your joy and that you can say "no." You know how much it can increase? You can say "no" even to God. That sounds like a joke to you, but it's true. Human history has recorded evidence when man said, "Ummm … no," and God agreed.

There was a king who got very uptight with Kabir.[24] He said, "I am going to mess this man up. He is a born Muslim, but he talks about Ram—which is Hindu—and he's messing me up." Kabir was sitting on a deer skin and meditating. So the king decided to tie him up with his deer skin, bundle him up, attach a huge stone boulder to it and ordered about two hundred men to carry it. That's how heavy it was. So they brought out the pulley and did the whole thing. They tied him up. The boulder was very heavy. And the king said "Dump him in the middle of the river."

The king was supervising and Kabir was dumped. There were millions of people watching. No bubbles came up. Nothing happened. They were very shocked. Finally they found the big boulder coming up the river and Kabir sitting on the deer skin, meditating. They couldn't believe it. Can you believe what happened to the king and everyone else? You can imagine it for yourself. The big boulder washed towards the shore. Kabir got off and put his deer skin on his back. People started touching the deer skin and him. He was wet because he was really in the river.

Some men have defied the law of nature because their nature has become the law. That is one who practices cross-reference. And that is your strength.

I was reading some notes about how every seven years a woman comes out to be new woman. She changes. Her consciousness changes—something like that. When she is seven years old, she wants to be married one day and have a family. It's a thought. When she is fourteen years old, she would like to have a man. At twenty-one years, she has a man. After twenty-eight years, she becomes a mother. She lives for the children. After another

---

[23] In Kundalini Yoga, there are cycles of life. The consciousness evolves every 7 years. The intelligence evolves every 11 years. And life, itself, goes into a new rhythm every 18 years.

[24] Kabir was a mystic poet, Sufi and yogi. He lived from 1440-1518. He was a predecessor of Guru Nanak. Many of Kabir's writings are included in the *Siri Guru Granth Sahib*.

seven years, she is for the family. The man comes in there somewhere—God knows where. So the man starts fighting, forgetting that he also changes every seven years. They call it the seven-year itch. Both get it.

If the woman knows that she was a woman first and the man knows he was a man first, and then they get married, then they become parents and then they become householders … if you just give the status its due, step by step, minute by minute, inch by inch, you will never suffer. If the duty is that of a woman, and the confrontation is that of a mother, deal with it as a woman first and a mother later.

Eighty percent of our children are ruined by their parents. Eighty percent. Because they give their children a long rope and a long leash. But time doesn't give it to them; society doesn't give it to them; nature doesn't give it to them; and so they live in misery.

I was dealing with parents one day and one of the parents was not willing to admit that there was anything wrong with their child. I said, "Come and see it." So we saw it together. Now understand this conversation.

The son said, "Hmm. You are my father. You have come to see me. Okay, dad, you have seen me. Now you can go back."

I said, "Wait a minute. This is your son?"

The father said, "Why is he doing this? He is not here. His body is here, but he is not here. What will happen?"

I said, "What will happen? One who cannot deal with his father as a father, how is he going to deal with a book as a book? How is he going to deal with life as life? How is is going to deal with food as food?"

Whenever you cannot face the reality of life, you switch gears. Either you get into your elementary nature and you get totally depressed; or you get into your professional identity, and become a total egomaniac; or you get into your fantasies and totally space out because you are three people. You are never one—you are a trinity. And if you don't have the cross-reference, and you don't have the capacity to have a cross fire to smooth yourself out of trouble, you will not make sense. It's very painful that your pain is both caused by you and faced by you.

The original power of a person is not ordinary. Whenever we believe that we are ordinary people, it's not true. We are very extraordinary. You all have a very unique power. It will stimulate in you your own uniqueness. It's not coming from outside. It's amazing that it can trigger things that you have never understood or done before.

Teach your children now all that you are learning, so when they grow, you may not have conflict with them. If you will become a teacher of your child, the relationship will be everlasting. If you become the parent of your child, after the first eighteen years you have to depart. The end will come. You have the natural right to be parents, but if you create the relationship between your child and you as a teacher and student, that relationship will last forever. Otherwise, every child has to become an adult by his or her own right. They have the right to walk out of the nest, which you don't like. But nobody denies the school of philosophy and love.

First, become a teacher to yourself. Then, the soul shall leave and be redeemed, in peace and tranquility and at one with God. If all of you become your own teacher, prosperity will be there. Good things will come to you. Good ideas will come to you because it's all in the magnetic framework of existence. All wisdom is within you. All knowledge is within you. All strength is within you. There is nothing you can get from outside. It simply has to be triggered. And to be very honest with you, that science to trigger the best in you is called Kundalini Yoga—small exercises, a couple of minutes. Human vitality is unlimited. It's Infinite. *Atman o paro purusham Paramatma naso satya. Atma* is just like that real God and it is true. You always use the power of your head and the power of your heart. Sometime, use the power of your soul. See what that can do.

Oh Designer, oh Maker, oh Guide, oh Guardian, oh Energy, oh Infinite, give this existence the peace, tranquility, honor and grace to understand and then to live in that understanding for happiness. Sat Nam.

> *All wisdom is within you.*
>
> *All knowledge is within you.*
>
> *All strength is within you.*
>
> *There is nothing you can get from outside.*
>
> *It simply has to be triggered.*

Chapter Seven

Know Your Defects

The alertness of your personality is based on three things: you are alert consciously, you are alert subconsciously and you are alert unconsciously. When you are alert, that does not mean you are awake. When you are alert, that does not mean you know. And when you are alert that does not mean you are truthful, or you are right, or any other positive thing. Alert does not mean all that. Alert only means three things: you are alert consciously, you are alert subconsciously and you are alert unconsciously. If these three states of mind are alert, then the person, personality and identity are alert, and such a person can assert happiness in life.

People are very corrupt. They go into middle age and they become a victim of a middle-age crisis. When they are poor, they are a victim of poverty. When they are rich, they are a victim of their wealth. If they are having sex they are a victim of their sexual life. No person is free and no person is a person by itself. You are all corrupt liars, momentary, and absolutely out-of-the-way human beings. You are not even supposed to be called a worm. There are billions of people on the earth who are victims of an emotion, a feeling, a projection, a dream, or a state of unconscious dream, conscious dream, subconscious dream.

God knows who you are. Nobody else knows who you are because you do not know who you are. When it is time to have sex, you axe it. When it is time to eat, you diet. When it is time to diet, you overeat. When it is time to be nice, you start throwing tantrums. When it is time to do a drama, you go silent. Everybody acts opposite to the environments in order

SUCCESS FORMULA FOR LEADERSHIP

Know the aim.

Know the fame.

You be you.

Pay attention to details.

Multiply your success.

to exert themselves. Among the animal kingdom you are known as God's shit. The birds call you that. The animals call you that. The underworld sea creatures and every life thinks you are God's poop. They can't understand you because your actions are absolutely illogical, irrational and unconventional to Mother Nature's actions and reactions.

Some of you are living the life of a mother. Some of you are living the life opposite of a mother. If a woman's father is very exact, and eternally good, and all that, she will end up with a totally neurotic ridiculous man. For a woman, you will absolutely find a man in your life who is opposite to the goodness of your father. And your father is always opposite to the goodness of his father.

So what are we doing? We are just yo-yo's. Our attitude is to live somebody else's life. What about our life? When is a person going to be alert and live one's own life? When is a person going to become what a person is going to be? God didn't make you to be a by-product of your mother and father. They were vehicles. How many times have you driven down the road and totally gotten lost in the scenery? Give me a break. Once you get lost in the scenery you will never make it. You are getting lost in the actions and reactions of your papa and mama and your neighbors. "My uncle tried to have intercourse with me and my father wanted to do me in and my uncle's brother—the same thing, and in school something happened." You know, you have stories. They were yesterday.

You are the most tragic living beings in history because you carry yesterday into tomorrow and you carry it today. Therefore you are useless, hopeless and tragic—these three things come to a human. If you could understand two birds talking and playing, you know what you would hear them say? "This idiot is a human but doesn't know a thing." That's what they say because you do not satisfy any emotional pattern. Do you know that? You humans who talk about emotions, feelings, consciousness, meditation and God knows what—religion and the whole thing—you are the supreme creation of God and you create wars. You kill everything in the world. You have done so much damage to this earth that the earth doesn't know what to do to itself. You have absolutely no feeling to follow the pattern of any emotions, and you have no idea how to follow the pattern of any idea. You are a bunch of insecure human beings who are trying to make things look good.

Your entire knowledge comes from what your father did to you, from what your mother did to you, from what your neighbor did to you. You have never decided to go inside and look at it. You have never decided to look at it as you, for you, within you, unto you. Do you understand?

Why is it that you cannot live as you? You have never tried to know who you are, really. You have never tried to know what your reality is. You have never tried to acknowledge your reality. And you have never tried to assert your reality.

You find every excuse in the book to be catered to. You want three things: you want to be catered to, you want to be acknowledged and you want to be paid attention to. That will never pay your bills. That will never cook your food, and you will always be raped. Anybody who can smell you out and understand you are insecure will attack you. If they cannot physically rape you, they will rape your psyche. If they cannot rape your psyche, they will insult you. If they cannot do anything, they will try to use and abuse you. They will make a football out of you. You will be part of football practice.

The only thing in life that is worthwhile is to be alert consciously, subconsciously, and unconsciously. You must know you are you. You must feel it. You must feel it and you must deal with it. You must play it and you must project it. If you think that the you within you is not important, that outside and inside are not important at all, you don't know a thing.

Husbands separate from wives. Wives separate from husbands. Men feel bad about women. Women feel bad about men. You know why? We conflict. Men don't know women, nor do women let the man know what his "you" is. You two end up barking like dogs and that's all we hear. "You told me this, you told me that, you told me . . ." You love to blame. You always love to blame. For twenty years I have counseled everybody. Everybody is so sick. All they tell me is that there is something else to be blamed because you never acknowledge yourself. Therefore you never blame yourself. Therefore you will never correct yourself. Therefore you can never be you.

ਕਬੀਰ ਸਭ ਤੇ ਹਮ ਬੁਰੇ ਹਮ ਤਜਿ ਭਲੋ ਸਭੁ ਕੋਇ ॥

Kabeer sabh tay ham buray ham taj bhalo sabh ko-ay.

Kabir says, "I am the worst of all. There is nobody worse than me."

— From *Siri Guru Granth Sahib*, page 1364, line 16,
as translated by Yogi Bhajan

If you do not know your worst, you do not know your best.

You are afraid to know your worst. First know your worst. Then know your best. Then keep the worst and go in the bathroom and flush it out. Take the best and give it to others, without asking for anything in return. If you ask for anything in return, you will get the other person's propositions and proposals; position and miseries; hidden and unhidden agendas. You will never be sovereign.

Whatever comes to you, put it on the altar, bow to it and be dedicated to it, including the sex and the husband. That is one thing a woman has to learn. Her approach to man is absolutely a simple approach. It is a gift from God. If the man is not a gift from God, life is a rift, rift, rift.

The human has only one escape—everything is a gift. All right—if it is not from God, it is from the unknown. If it is not from the unknown, call it something, anything. Life is a gift because prana is a gift. So whatever sustains your prana has to be a gift. Otherwise, within your surroundings, within you and over you, above you, below you, to the right of you, to the left of you—there will be nothing but a rift. There will be no goodness but a gulf. You will be totally drowned in your own negativity. You don't need an enemy. You don't need to call the neighbors to make you miserable. You are miserable by your own right.

So therefore, please learn to be creative and know your defects first. De-facts. If you want the facts, first know the de-facts. When you know the de-facts then find out how the de-facts keep you away from defects. Nobody keeps you away from the facts of your own defects. The only way that you can have self-consciousness, self-acknowledgement and self-respect is that you must totally, privately and personally verify your defects. Find out how you are kept away from the facts. Once you find where the facts are, they are yours. This is a very simple lifestyle. Before people find your defects and embarrass you, before people find your defects and harass you, before people find your defects and make you miserable, find your own defects. Then, you can be absolutely strong and capable of handling, facing and confronting them.

> *Fact your de-facts.*
>
> *Life will be free, happy, conscious and absolutely enjoyable.*

If you do not want to be a victim, you must be victorious. There is no alternative to life. Either be a victim or be victorious. If you want to be victorious, you must know your defects before they get to you. If you do not know them, you cannot defend yourself.

Self-knowledge is not knowing how long of a nose you have. Self-knowledge is knowing how many defects you have and to what degree—impulsively, emotionally, consciously, unconsciously and subconsciously—they keep you away from your factual life. Fact your de-facts. Life will be free, happy, conscious and absolutely enjoyable.

There is no rhythm in life that you can get through counseling or by religion. This *Raj Yog*[25], this golden link of Guru Ram Das, provides a very safe clue to it.

Man has the right to go to the depth of a ditch from which he can't jump out. It is called self-pit, self-pity. When you put your self into the pit, you experience self-pity and self-pity is one of the biggest diseases. Once a person gets into self-pity, that person is totally ruined. It is quicksand. The more you try to come out of it, the deeper you go. Medical science can give you B-complex and other things, but that lasts only for a short time. Then you start having side effects.

What I am trying to do is to set a pattern in which adversity, calamity and tragedy becomes a game for the people who believe in God. There is no possibility that things won't go wrong. What I am saying is, we want to produce people who, in a few generations, can sing songs in the face of things going wrong. People who won't vanish. Who become victorious. It doesn't take much. It only takes mental grit. You must understand, when you want to do something, you have to put your identity into it. It's not that work must identify with you. You must identify into the work. Then, you become the nucleus of the identity of that work and you will succeed. If you will not do that, then you will fail. Failure and success are just very little things.

It isn't the life that matters. It's the courage you bring to it.

---

[25] *Raj Yog* – Royal Yoga. Where perfect spirituality and absolutely royal living merge into one existence.

**FIVE ASPECTS TO COMPUTE
AND CONSIDER**

Whenever I do something,
I ask myself:

Will it exalt me?

Will it show my excellence?

Will it prove I am a human?

Would I like this to happen to me?

And finally, within my best
knowledge, is it the best I can do?

CHAPTER EIGHT

APPLY THE WISDOM

Editor's Note: The following lecture is an excerpt from a talk given by the Siri Singh Sahib to the International Khalsa Council. The International Khalsa Council is a leadership body created by the Siri Singh Sahib comprised of long-standing teachers and ministers involved in Sikh Dharma International.

All the knowledge you have, you have. You have a lot of knowledge. Practical wisdom. I call it, "Applied wisdom." If you just share your applied wisdom with people—without considering that you have to influence or acquire something and without requiring something—you will have masses of people loving you and following you, because you are very unique people.

We have come from the sixties and that revolt was very costly. There were twenty million people in America who started the revolt. It was an honest, constitutional revolt. Today, the sixties rule the United States. And if we are not aware of that, we are highly handicapped.

You are the by-product of the evolution of the United States of America. You went through it and this evolution will affect this country for the coming 5,000 years. America will never be the same again and you are the cream of that. Like white butter coming out of milk.

A lot of people died. They OD'd. It was an evolution in the shape of a revolution. People revolted. People discussed. People challenged. And then they mellowed and then they merged. Out of that merger, we find a class by itself. An absolutely classic class by itself merged to become *Sikh Dharma* of the Western Hemisphere.[26] And it organized itself. It grew into a cohesive body of intellectual, intelligent and practically committed people. You live it. And that's a very powerful, unique experience. It's a practical acknowledgement. So I am not unhappy with what is happening.

Now, in the last twenty years, do you think there were earthquakes? There were, right? Tidal waves? Hurricanes? Storms? Twisters? Count them all. We didn't experience THAT much tragedy. Though we were hit by twisters. We were hit by tidal waves. We had earthquakes. That's what happened. We had a very powerful lobby conspiring to see that we would disintegrate.

I'll tell you a law of physics. If an existence comes into existence that does not merge itself into the existence, it always takes over the total existence. This is a law that can never change. If your existence continues to be identified as it is—complete, in spite of a little cheating here and there. I'm not saying 100%, but if it could have been 100%. Just your existence—as it is in *bana, bani, seva, simran*[27]—continues, and as you pass this on from one generation to another generation to another generation to another generation, do you know that the entire vicinity and the entire force of life will be forced by the law of physics, by the laws of nature, to start merging with you and multiplying with you, without you asking.

FORMULA FOR HAPPINESS

Commitment will give you character.

Character will give you dignity.

Dignity will give you divinity.

Divinity will give you grace.

Grace will give you the power to sacrifice.

Power to sacrifice will give you happiness.

Where you are, you are valuable but comparatively comfortable. You have problems. You have solutions, too. But you do not apply the solution to your problems. The only time a person cannot solve his problems is when he cannot sacrifice. Remember this law. Every problem needs a solution. The problem will not go away. Every problem needs a solution and every solution needs a sacrifice. And every sacrifice will bring harmony. When you buy something, you pay in dollars. When you buy happiness, you pay through sacrifice.

Nobody has achieved infinity, grace and tranquility within his own component units without sacrificing one thing: his commotional concept before his identification.

---

[26] In later years, the name of the organization changed to Sikh Dharma International.
[27] Four pillars of Sikh Dharma. *bana*: a code of dressing that includes wearing a turban; *bani*: reciting the sacred songs of Guru Nanak and the other masters from the Sikh tradition; *seva*: selfless service; *simran*: deep meditation to connect the mind and the spirit.

I'm not saying that you do not have the right to feel or that you do not have the right to think, or that you do not have the right to be. But one right you do not have. With all the knowledge from thinking, feeling, emotions, commotions, desire, responsibility and understanding, there is one right you don't have: you cannot act against your own identity. If you ever let yourself act against your own identity, you are your own worst enemy. Please understand this simple secret of totality.

The question was asked yesterday evening during a discussion, "How can the Infinite God become a slave to the finite man?" It was a direct question. The reply that I shared with that person, I will share with you. When a simple, humble, mortal man starts believing, trusting and loving his identity over and above his feelings, his emotions, thoughts and ideas, at that time the Infinity of God becomes the Infinity of the man. And because of that beauty and success, God surrenders Itself to the very little tiny man we call human.

That's the only process available in this universe. That's why from human beings we become the Sikhs, and from the Sikhs we become the *Khalsa*. Then we live to the purity of it, to the end of it, so that we can be free from beginning to end, once and for all. Life has two attitudes. One is you live for the sake of yourself. *Nit nam. Namit. Namit* is "for the sake of." Nit is "daily." You live your daily life as daily life. Or you live for the sake of the *Guru*.

If you decide to live each day of yours for the sake of the *Guru*, then God shall live for you forever. That's how ordinary people born in an ordinary way of life become holy and become messengers and messiahs.

The point of termination is the point of determination. When your determination becomes complete, your negativity terminates before you. All the problems in our lives are because we don't have determination. Termination of negativity, weakness, cowardice and shallowness is only experienced when the determination of identity, personality and reality through the identity are objectively known.

One day I'll be physically gone. I'll be better off gone than being here. But, it is no secret to my mind and to my heart that there are many of you, all of you or some of you—I'm not getting into numbers—whose prayer has drawn a triangle over the square of God's order of death.

In my own experience, lying on the surgical table, I experienced death for a second time in my life. I was gone. But when I heard the shout of the doctor, "Yogiji, Yogiji!" I also heard the chanting and prayers of all of you, too. I apologized to the doctor for answering him a little later than I should have.

He said, "Are you here? Are you okay?"

"I am fine. I am enjoying myself. Don't worry about it."

"What?"

"Well, you don't know. Go ahead. I am okay, now."

After that, my entire circulatory system collapsed because it clotted. I have never felt such a burning sensation in my entire chest. It felt like I was on a hot plate—on fire. Being roasted.

Then I said, "Actually, there is something wrong."

They took me back again and did the whole surgery. But it was fine. It was fun. It was over.

What I am trying to explain to you is that many of you may not recognize your identity, your power, your spirituality and your realism. But you have that graciousness.

The only purpose of life is not to be scared of insecurity. Insecurity does nothing but scare a person. It's a scarecrow. It is a scarecrow that will not let opportunity and grace come and sit and be friendly. Listen—whatever is going to happen is going to happen. There's nothing anybody can do. If you feel insecure about it, bad things WILL happen. If you don't feel insecure, they go away. That's the Catch-22.

The purpose of prayer is to tie in with Infinity. It's simple mathematics. The purpose of prayer is to tie into Infinity and when a zero ties into Infinity, it becomes Infinity. Infinity means "all powerful." That just means you are not scared, you are not afraid. That's all it means. You project your fear through prayer with Infinity and multiply and tune in—and your fear goes away. When your fear goes away, the divine takes over.

Fear and divinity do not live together. That's why in the entire *Siri Guru Granth Sahib,* they say if you are afraid, be afraid of God. Any fear of God is no fear. It is a reverence. In the western mind, fear is a very dreadful thing. In the eastern mind, fear is a reverence. When you are afraid of somebody, you have reverence about it.

To me, it is about *Bhao* and *Bhaao.* Fear (*Bhao*) creates reverence (*Bhaao*). When I go to the Gurdwara[28], I am afraid that I will do something wrong, so I am very self-contained. I have complete reverence and command over myself. When I bow to the *Guru*[29], I have a great reverence for the *Guru.* Now *Guru* is not sitting there, pulling my ears or doing something to me. But I have a great reverence because I am afraid if I misbehave in the presence of my *Guru,* it will be wrong.

The fear that is being afraid to act wrong gives you reverence. You do not know what reverence is. You think that if you can insult somebody—emotionally, commotionally, speak it all out—that you have reverence. No, that's not reverence. That is called unloading what you couldn't unload in the bathroom.

You have factories and situations where the unloading and loading department is always separate. Do you know that? You may build a million-dollar house, but you cannot have an outhouse with it. That becomes an inside issue.

Yesterday, somebody was telling me about a house that is available—five bedrooms, and five and a half bathrooms. I said, "What is beautiful about it?"

He said, "There's a half bathroom more."

"What is the beauty of that?"

"The moment you enter, the closet is like a living room. There is a half bathroom there so the guest can ease himself."

"That's a new idea."

So there is a half bathroom available right away. You take your shoes off, and put your coat on a hanger and there's a mirror and there's a place to wash and then there's a bathroom so you are all set—groomed. But if a man comes to a five million-dollar house and he has to use an outhouse, will you be lucky enough that he will visit you a second time?

---

[28] *Gurdwara:* Sikh temple.
[29] In the Sikh *Gurdwara,* the *Siri Guru Granth Sahib* presides. When Sikhs come into the temple, they bow to the *Siri Guru Granth Sahib* as their living Guru, the *Shabad Guru.*

When you unload yourself in public, it is just like unloading yourself in the living room and not in the bathroom. I call it mis-management of the brain wavelength of a personality not to relate to the decor of the environmental institution of authoritative replacement. Because when you misbehave publicly, unload yourself publicly, you may feel that you are very truthful, but you are not. In spite of the fact that you may be truthful, really you are mannerless.

Three things are very important for a man to progress: reverence, manners and kindness. Reverence, manners and kindness. When these three things become your mode of life, then compassion comes. Compassion gives you three things. Compassion for people will give you the authority over your own passions. Compassion for others gives you the authority to relate to the reality of others. Compassion gives you the authority to gain other people's trust without even asking for it.

Therefore in the decor of the human, one can be highly decorated if one understands that compassion is the key to success. Intellectually, if you are compassionate, you can put yourself in the other person's position and totally understand their psyche. Therefore you will not have any confrontations. You can avoid those issues.

So in my realism, I feel that the future holds a very bright and promising, graceful time for those who will continue to serve Sikh Dharma and the Khalsa unity with their own integrity, identity and self on the line.

It is my very beautiful experience that if there is a challenge you should start finding a solution. Don't waste your time in challenging a challenge. The greatest challenge to a challenge is to find the solution. It is in my brightest feeling that God has,

ਜੋ ਕਿਛੁ ਪਾਇਆ ਸੁ ਏਕਾ ਵਾਰ ॥
Jo kichh paa-i-aa so aykaa vaar.

God has given us all that He wanted to give us once.

— Guru Nanak, *Japji Sahib*, Pauree 31, as translated by Yogi Bhajan

We can use it as we want. When we start using things gracefully, they multiply for us. The grace extends happiness in our life. The graceful attitude determines happiness.

You can very well take my personal example. I came here twenty years ago, I never knew which boulevard, which country or which city I was going to. I wandered—a man without direction. But I knew God was asking me to come here, so there was a purpose.

I went to the university saying, "I am supposed to be teaching in the university."[30] They said, "Well, I don't know what will happen, but we can start your classes under the engineering department." Now how do yoga and engineering go together?

I said, "What does yoga have to do with the engineering department?"

"Well, there are funds available in engineering more than in any other department."

"Is there a philosophy department?"

"They are all under-funded."

[30] Yogi Bhajan came from India to the West in the late 1960s when a university in Canada invited him to teach yoga there.

So under the engineering department I started teaching Kundalini Yoga. Can you believe that? I didn't believe it myself, but it happened. And it only could happen in Canada—nowhere else. My realization was, "Wow, look at this."

Then, when I came to America, there were many, many opportunities—bright and beautiful offers. There was once an opportunity that I would not have to raise my pinkie for the rest of my life. I could just sit. It was suggested that the funds were so much, I could advertise on every billboard in every city in the United States. They even suggested that I have a huge picture of myself telling them, "I am, I am." All I had to do was put my little hand on this little lady's head and say, "I initiate you."

I said, "No. In Kundalini Yoga, nobody initiates anybody." She said, "Why not?" I said, "If a man or a woman is not worthy enough to initiate himself or herself, the law of Kundalini Yoga is that person should not be taught. I'm not going to flout that law."

> *This is the yoga to guarantee that you'll be happy. It guarantees you. There's a divine promise. It's a divine guarantee to make you healthy, happy and holy. Provided you initiate yourself into it.*

This is the yoga to guarantee that you'll be happy. It guarantees you. There's a divine promise. It's a divine guarantee to make you healthy, happy and holy. Provided you initiate yourself into it. This is the only yoga that has a pre-requisite of self-initiation. It says from self-initiation to self-enlightenment, the path is guaranteed. You have been practicing it for the last twenty years, nineteen years, eighteen years, fifteen years, twelve years. You are on the right path. It may not be absolutely perfect. The progress may not be right, according to you, because you assess it incorrectly.

Look at the assessment the way I look at it. Who are you? You were a commoner. Now you are special. You were a commoner with common weaknesses. Now, at least, you are a special looking person with a common weakness. Although you practice those common weaknesses the fact is that you know they are common weaknesses.

People are very afraid of being lonely. They are extremely afraid to be lonely. The luckiest thing is to be lonely. There's no higher experience of Infinity and divinity bestowed but to be lonely—because God is lonely.

There's only One God. We don't see a second, so who will He do it with? Name the person. God is very lonely—extremely lonely. Because when you are lonely, you are forced to be self-fulfilled. There's an automatic process in it. Self-fulfillment only comes when you become lonely. Self-degradation and self-inferiority hit you only when you are lonely. You have the right to life, therefore you challenge that loneliness, and what it brings to you. From that you start creating a society.

For a teacher, it is a factual fact that he has to be lonely. From that loneliness he gets tired like God. And God created the universe. Therefore a teacher, when he starts feeling lonely, and starts getting depressed with loneliness, at that time he'll start teaching more classes. Believe me or not.

All weirdos become great teachers. All great teachers are basically those weirdos who never wanted to be lonely but they have no option but to be lonely. So they create like kind. It is called "twin intercourse."

If you look at the life of all great people whom you call special incarnations of God, their life stories will be based on twin intercourse. Their mental psyche explored the balance of their physical existence and their spiritual exaltedness. The human body is exactly curved, cut and made with an idea to have that experience.

In a spiritual twilight when you exist in the light of your own soul's spirit, in the guidance of your own spirit, in your own spiritual twilight zone, then God seeks you. You don't have to seek God. And to enter into your own spiritual twilight zone, you have to have a twin intercourse with your own soul. Your identity and your soul relate to each other in a dialog, in an understanding, in a flow, and that establishes the frequency that creates the magnetic field through which the attractiveness is not fatal, but fortunate. There can be fatal attractions but there can also be fortunate attractions. And it is that fortunate attraction that brings you prosperity, happiness, love of friends, glory of God and understanding with the mother earth and the Universe.

Honorable members of this council, wisdom and knowledge are the beauties that I—in my humble opportunity of the grace of God—work to understand. I have three things to count on. One: I experienced that I served my teacher flawlessly. You have a magnitude and attitude about service. Let me tell you my own experience and I'm not telling you what's right or wrong. I might have done certain wrong things or right things in my innocence, or in my coveting, whatever you want to call it. But all error is human. It's no big deal. Yet in one thing I found myself to be very honest within myself. I served my teacher flawlessly, and that was a very graceful experience.

Then—I served my *Guru* very humbly. Extremely humbly. Because when I was posted at Amritsar[31], the only job that I loved and liked and looked forward to was mopping up the floors of the *parkarma*.[32] That was my second experience. I served my teacher who gave me the knowledge, basic knowledge, flawlessly. And I served the *Guru* very humbly. And third: I served any office given to me, with the utmost dedication, with utmost reverence. Wherever I got posted, I used to say to the people, "Look, I don't know what I am, but I'll do everything to serve this office in which I am."

That's why I developed a habit to ask opinions. One day I was asking an opinion from my doorman. One of my inspectors came by and said, "My God, why are you asking the doorman?"

[31] Before coming to the West, Yogi Bhajan served the government of India. At one point, he was stationed in the city of Amritsar. The city of Amritsar was founded by Guru Ram Das and is the home of the Harimandir Sahib or Golden Temple, which is the most sacred temple in the Sikh faith.
[32] The Golden Temple is in the middle of a pool of water. Surrounding the water on all sides is a large marble walkway called the **parkarma**. Every night, people volunteer to clean the *parkarma*. This is open to anyone who wants to participate.

I said, "He met that man first. I want his impression before I make mine." He was a very ordinary doorman standing at my door. This man must not have hidden his personality at all when he passed him. With me he might have hidden his personality. So, pick up knowledge from everywhere and anywhere and use it.

There are two ways to decide things: the inductive method and the deductive method. Deduce things to come to conclusions and also induce the environment to see whether what you deduce fits in. Otherwise, there is a possibility that your decisions will be wrong. You have to develop "automation" in you. Automatically when you induce things, you should deduce the result. And when you deduce the result, the environments should induce to second your deductive results. When you start thinking and inducing and deducing things, actually you are learning to become intuitive. Whenever you'll decide everything inducively and deducively, you will become intuitively self-plus and then surplus. Once you become surplus in your intuition, you have the day. There's nothing to it.

CHAPTER NINE

GET RID OF YOUR "COULDN'T"

In our life there are three difficult things: the first is to pass our time, the second is to know our tomorrow and the third is to meet our obligations—which are a demand on us. That's the process of life. Most of the time we cannot save ourselves from our emotions. When we cannot save ourselves from our emotions, we cannot use our intuition, so we are not aware of our tomorrow. That's why a guide becomes necessary. Otherwise there is no necessity for a man to have a guide. We are very fortunate that, with the *Shabad Guru* of the *Siri Guru Granth Sahib*, there are fourteen hundred and thirty pages, that are nothing but guidance. And it all comes to one understanding. There is no heaven and there is no hell. There is no guilt and there is no nonsense. All you have to do is to make sense. To whom? To yourself. But we try to make sense to everybody else except ourselves. Therefore, we are victims of our own concept. We are victims of our attachment. We are victims of our greed. We are victims of our anger, etcetera, etcetera. Because basically, all these things makes us handicapped.

A child is born with your own blood and with your blood money you raise that child. You want to give your child values and virtues. Is that true?

On the other hand, you also want to mold the child in your concept. So there is a destiny and there is you. Similarly, there is a destiny and there is you for you. There is a child in you, too. And you want to mold the child the way you want it, not as destiny wants. So you have no freedom from yourself.

For the last twenty to thirty years I have been counseling people. They tell me their story. I listen to the story. It all comes down to two things: how the father behaved and how the mother behaved. That's it. And when I tell them the father and mother are not here, it is you who are here, do you know what they say to me? "I don't know how to do it."

In one case, the father passed away twenty-five years ago. The mother passed away fifteen years ago. The guy is still struggling. Now, in turn, he wants to behave the same way with his children and raise the children to his concept. I said to him, "In ten or twenty years you will not be there. What will happen to your child?"

He wants me to help. For their whole lives, the children have been made phobic. Now he needs my help? Why? I told him, "You made them phobic. You make them unphobic. You told them not to go out. You told them not to do this. You told them this and that. You have been constantly cluckling at them like crazy. Now, you want a psychologist-sociologist-personal trainer for them? It can't work. It can't work."

You know, I have seen colleagues in my life who used to take huge bundles of files home. You know, in my whole life, I have not taken one file, one paper home?

They would ask me, "How did you do it?"

I said, "What is there to do? This is the office. That is home. What relates to my office, I deal with it here. What relates to my home, I deal with it there. I am not going to take my office home or bring my home to the office."

I used to go home and take off my uniform and that was the end of it. Hallelujah, there's nothing else. I would get up in the morning, get ready, everything would be shining and glittering and I would go to the office. That's the office. They were two different lives. And you have two options in life: either you are on top of your business or you are in the bottom of your business. Choose which way you want it.

Life is a conception. Why do you want to twist it? There is nothing that will not test your guts. So what is the conclusion about life? The conclusion about life is one thing and one thing only: either you compromise with your grace or you don't. And whether you compromise with your grace or not, do you do it for your own sake and not for somebody else's? Not somebody else's. That's the trouble we have when our children become twenty-one, eighteen, fifteen, seventeen, twenty-two, twenty-three. They rebel. Because they have not been taught the truth. They have been forced to swallow it.

You marry your wife. On the very first day of the honeymoon, you start being a control freak—on the very first day.

You know where the problem happens? When a man organizes their life and he subconsciously runs it and she doesn't know it. And when she realizes it, she takes a chile and puts it in his ass and there is not one psychiatrist, psychologist or religious priest, who can save that marriage. Not one.

The vengeance of a woman is so powerful. People saw God running once and they looked around to see what was making Him run. There was a woman with a fireball chasing after Him. Woman is made with the capacity of being a mother, of being lovely, of being nice, the whole story. But when she finds it out that she has been cheated, then watch out. The comedy turns into a tragedy to that extent that you can't even believe it.

Woman can give birth. She can turn her blood into milk. She can make love. She can keep the house absolutely calm, quiet and peaceful. She can tolerate a man's nonsense. All of this is true.

But on the other hand, everything has an equal and opposite side to it. The same woman can be a disastrous, murderous planner and she can cut the roots of the man—the same woman. It depends on which channel you're working. That's the truth.

If you just treat her like a woman and she treats you like a man, there cannot be a conflict. If you treat a child as a child and when the child becomes an adult, you treat him or her as an adult and not a child, then there can't be a conflict. It is up to you. Because there is no such thing as God outside of you. When you close these eyes forever, your God closes His eyes forever. You have no participation in it. Your God starts with you, goes with you and ends with you. But you can't live that way. You have guilt. You have been told to carry one and a half tons of guilt at least. So you can never be you. You can never be you.

So what do you have to do? You have to save yourself from yourself. You have to drop that guilt. That's why we are a community. That's why we are a family. That's why we are together. We can get it together. You will never find a community leader who doesn't know how to give. *Seva.*[33] Giving is the only way. Don't only give to those who ask. Give to those who don't ask. Keep on giving. Become a giver. Your faculty and God's faculty will become the same. That's divinity—absolute divinity.

ਦੇਦਾ ਦੇ ਲੈਦੇ ਥਕਿ ਪਾਹਿ ॥

Daydaa day laiday thak paahi.

You, Great Giver, keep giving to us and we grow tired of just taking.

— Guru Nanak, *Japji Sahib*, Pauree 3

You should be so conscious and so giving that people get tired of your hospitality.

Some people have never had the chance to sit together with another person and eat. How often, out of joy, have you forced other people to break bread with you? How many times was somebody eating and you had the guts to sit with that person and start eating from the same plate? And you call yourself human?

God and divinity and nonsense and all the yak-yak claims and yoga and standing on your head and everything. What is it? What you have learned? How many people have you hugged? How many children you have played with? You are looking for romance and you

---

[33] *Seva:* sefless service.

don't have any romance with nature, the *prakriti*? What are you up to? In this life there are challenges. These challenges challenge how much sweetness is in you and how much that sweetness you want to share.

There is one God, one God—that idiot God who still takes care of you in spite of the fact you don't deserve it. That one God. How many times have you become one with each other in the name of God? How much nearness have you created? How relaxed are you when somebody makes a mistake? Where is your kindness and compassion?

There is a university called the universe. There is a great teacher in this university called nature. There is a great subject called the faculty of life. We want to give our children that freedom so it can become their choice.

You have to walk on your own two legs. That's the challenge of life. Today or tomorrow or the day after or twenty years from now, you have to walk. You have to face this world.

When I was in Alaska, I went to the house of a student. They lived in a home by the creek and I said to his wife, "Do you know what is happening on the planet?"

She said, "It is revolving."

That was the answer. She said, "It is revolving. It creates a day and night for me. How can I forget that Yogiji?"

I said, "You are the best in the world."

It's very funny how people understand life—climatically, critically and complainingly. But there is one class of people who are complimenting. They have no attachment. They compliment their Creator. They are grateful.

Creative supplement is required for life to grow in peace and tranquility. And a consistent sense of radiance of the Tenth Body[34] is required to protect us. The Subtle Body must give us our intuitive self so that we can understand what is coming to us. Every day we should socialize and be kind to each other to grow our ultimate aura. If somebody has fallen, we should raise that person up. If somebody is going down, we should lift him. If somebody is hungry, we should feed him. If somebody is unhappy we should dance with him. There are things to do and those things are part of us.

Somebody once asked me, "Is it really important to go to your class? Is it a must?"

I said, "Yes."

"Why?"

"Well, I have beautiful students, don't worry. Simply, you are reminded every time you see them that you are gracious and not guilty. It's worth your few bucks."

"Why?"

I said, "Why do you get a massage?"

"I relax."

"Well, go to my class and you will relax. Because you will be told that the subconscious tension you create, the subconscious fear you create, the subconscious being you create is unwanted. It is not required."

---

[34] In the teachings shared by Yogi Bhajan, a human has ten bodies. First is the Soul. Second is the Negative Mind. Third is the Positive Mind. Fourth is the Neutral Mind. Fifth is the Physical Body. Sixth is the Arcline—the power of prayer. Seventh is the Aura. Eighth is the Pranic Body—the body relating to breath. Ninth is the Subtle Body. Tenth is the Radiant Body. When all of these bodies work together consciously, it creates the Eleventh Body—the Perfected Body.

That's one way to be happy. To serve people who share divinity, who allow us to accumulate our integrity, who give us a moment of grace. This life is a real thing.

Life is like a beautiful, beautiful, marvelous horse but you are crippled riding it. You have unnecessary problems, unnecessary attachments, unnecessary things and then you believe that God does everything. If God does everything what are you bothered about? Because you cannot believe it—you cannot trust it. He gives you the breath of life and you create a commentary with it.

Have you seen football, baseball—whatever they play? There is a box up there. Some people sit there and they comment on the players, right? They don't play. They are not in the field. They are sitting on the top of the universe, "Oh, he did this, he did that." That's what you do.

You do not guide your ego to the strength of straightforwardness. You just comment on everything and create a drama.

And what do we do at home when we are listening to the television? "Oohhhh… he hit so good. Come on boy. Run after it." Have you seen people watching a game at home? Thank God they don't break the TV screens. They are into it like they are the ones who are playing. When the game is over, they are still in their living home. They didn't go anywhere.

One person was watching a game. When the game stopped, he ran to bathroom.

I said, "Why didn't you get up sooner?"

He said, "It was during the game."

He wanted to go urinate for that whole time, and he stopped it. That is how much you can get involved in maya. You know it is not real, but you feel it is real. Why not feel the real as real?

One man was sitting once. He had an earthen pot with a plant in it. His wife said, "Come inside."

He said, "Just wait. I am coming."

After one hour she came out and said, "What's going on? You are looking at this plant and this vase. What is in it?"

"Don't disturb me. I am coming."

After an hour she brought a big stick and she said, "Are you coming in or I am going to break this plant and break this vase and everything."

"Why?"

"You have been staring at it for two hours. What are you looking at?"

"Come sit with me."

She sat down. He said, "See that branch? That little branch—that little one."

"Yes, I see that branch. What is it?'

"There is a little leaf coming out of it. Just watch, watch, watch."

"Where?"

"Just watch, don't yell. The leaf will be hurt. Just watch. The branch is sprouting with a little leaf."

"Well, they all do it. Just come in."

He said, "No I am watching. You watch with me."

But there was no oneness. There was no sophistication. There was no togetherness. There was no reality. For him it was the greatest dawn of the universe to see a little leaf coming out of the little bud on the branch. For his wife it was impossible because dinner was getting cold, the sun was setting and he was wasting his time. That's where we conflict.

Our reach to the nature, the *prakriti*, is different.

What we get out of our holiness is intuition. We can see in time what shall be. The sequence has started, and we can see what the consequences shall be. But when we are not with the flow, we do not know.

> *We want to make our will so clean, so clear, so positive, that the "couldn't" doesn't touch our shores.*

That's why, sometimes, I sit like this and we repeat a few words. Then we meditate[35] for a few minutes. Because when we sit collectively, and meditate collectively, the total sum of that experience purifies our being.

Do you remember a day when you wanted to come to class and you couldn't? It happens. It happens many times. It happens when you wanted to get up in the morning and be with your God and lord, but you couldn't. It happens when you wanted to love somebody and serve somebody. You really wanted to do it but you couldn't. We want to get rid of this "couldn't." We want to make our will so clean, so clear, so positive, that the "couldn't" doesn't touch our shores. We have a very strong disease. It's called "couldn't." And ultimately this couldn't is like a cancer. It eats our *pratigya*—our determination, our essence—because we "couldn't."

All our problems on this planet come from this "couldn't." This "couldn't" makes us slip from our *dharma*, from our duty.

Just imagine Guru Gobind Singh, the tenth master. He had to decorate his younger son, himself, and send him to war.[36] He could do it and he did it. Because he had a mastery over "couldn't." The Sikhs were there. They said, "Lord, you are not supposed to send your son until we are finished."

He said, "No, let him go and face the war."

For the sake of the glory of the *dharma*, Guru Gobind Singh decorated his own sons to go into war where one hundred twenty-five thousand people per one Sikh solider were fighting.

Reality has reverence and there is nothing else. Because this life—this one life—is given to us for completion.

When I came to United States and I started teaching Kundalini Yoga, I knew at least that it is a science that gives a person excellence. It will create excellent characters. It will take away the "couldn't." It will give us a pathway of essential sacrifice—which will give us

---

[35] In the meditation section: Get Rid of Your Couldn't. 9/4/01
[36] At the Battle of Chamkaur Sahib in 1704, Guru Gobind Singh's two eldest sons, Baba Ajit Singh and Baba Jujhar Singh, fought bravely against the Mughal armies and died. They were 17 and 15 years old respectively.

maximum happiness. We cannot sacrifice our ego. We cannot sacrifice our attachment. We cannot sacrifice our anger. We cannot sacrifice our lust. We cannot sacrifice our greed. Then, what can we sacrifice? These are the faculties that force our "couldn't" on us.

We make every effort to survive. But we need to survive with the ultimate reality, with applied consciousness, and with absolute reality of grace. We can't compromise. Some people can do it. Some can't. There's nothing personal in it. You can live like a frog in the well or you can live in the ocean. It's up to you. Things will not change if you don't change them. And what will change things in you is that You—the divine You—which is in you. It is the divinity in you that will allow you to sacrifice. It is the reality in you that will bring you realization. Don't take it personally. It is not personal. It's a general rule of *prakriti*. It is the law of the lord. *Purkha* and *prakriti*. It shall never change. You have to change with it.

Baba Deep Singh was seventy-two years old. He had two hundred and fifty people. They were ten miles away from Amritsar. He drew the line and said, "Those who have the willingness to go, come along with me now. Those who have the determination to go, cross this line." Fortunately, everybody crossed. With two hundred and fifty people he attacked a hundred thousand men—fully trained—to liberate the Golden Temple.[37] When he got beheaded in an attack along with the commander of the enemy forces, somebody reminded him, "You took a vow that you won't die until your head bows at the temple." This event is recorded by enemy sources. It is not a made-up story.

Baba Deep Singh said, "Pick up my head and put it in my left hand,"

The soldier obeyed. Baba Deep Singh stood up, with his head in his left hand, and started fighting again. The enemy forces ran—they had never seen such a phenomena.

These are human powers. They met the challenge of *prakriti* and defied it for their purpose. That's called commitment. That gives you character. That gives you dignity, divinity, grace, the power to sacrifice and then happiness. Because the only thing that dies is the physical body. But there are nine other bodies. The total account is ten bodies. That's the reality. You have to learn to love all the ten bodies, not only your physical body. Even if you don't destroy the physical body, it is going to destroy itself. That's the law of *prakriti*.

ਜੋ ਉਪਜਿਓ ਸੋ ਬਿਨਸਿ ਹੈ ਪਰੋ ਆਜੁ ਕੈ ਕਾਲਿ ॥

Jo upji-o so binas hai paro aaj kai kaal.

Whatever has been created shall be destroyed; everyone shall perish, today or tomorrow.

— Guru Teg Bahadur, *Siri Guru Granth Sahib*,
page 1429, line 4

One who is born has to die. But the other bodies can help you be young, fresh and beautiful. This body is given to serve and to recognize that there are nine other bodies with it. That is called the path of *dharma*. And it is up to you to follow it or deny it.

---

[37] In 1755-56, warriors from Afghanistan raided India and annexed the Punjab region. They controlled the complex of the Harimandir Sahib and fouled the waters around the temple. In 1757, Baba Deep Singh called for a group of Sikhs a go with him and reclaim the Harimandir Sahib.

Life is to be lived. Life is a given gift. *Atma*, the soul, takes the body. The distance of life is covered by destiny and challenged by fate. That's how it goes. There are no two ways about it.

There are some people who live life by making their security just the earth—the here and now. They box themselves in. They feel insecure. They feel irrelevant to the environments if they are not secure. And their security is very important to them. So they box themselves in and it's kind of a prison.

Whereas *atma*, the pranic *shakti*[38], is also a prisoner of the ribcage. It breathes in and out. It can go in and out. But when a person with his ego boxes himself in because of his insecurity, then there's no place to go in and out. Then a person goes deeper and deeper, layer by layer, and enslave's one's atma—one's self. Then that person does not have any sensitivity to feel others. All they want to know is whether or not their security is secure.

Now, there are other people who live a life of mission. They live a life to love everybody. They are smiling. They are beautiful. They support everybody.

ਹਰਿ ਕਾ ਨਾਮੁ ਧਿਆਇ ਕੈ ਹੋਹੁ ਹਰਿਆ ਭਾਈ ॥
ਕਰਮਿ ਲਿਖੰਤੈ ਪਾਈਐ ਇਹ ਰੁਤਿ ਸੁਹਾਈ ॥

Har kaa naam Dhi-aa-ay kai hohu hari-aa bhaa-ee.
Karam likhantai paa-ee-ai ih rut suhaa-ee.

Take the Name of the Creator God and be healthy. Opportunities will come.

— Guru Arjan Dev Ji, *Siri Guru Granth Sahib*, page 1193, line 7, as translated by Yogi Bhajan

You know, you have your life. You can live. You can have all that you need, and that is destined. But if you want more, you can only get it if you open yourself. Open your doors. A person has to open his heart to others. It is not necessary to try to predominate or dominate other people. Your one beautiful smile, and one, "Hello, how are you?" or "Sat Nam,"—there is so much good it can do, even to a person who doesn't know you. But to do that, you have to put in your investment. You have to move towards the psyche of another person. You have to show that you are the beloved of the Lord and you are here to live a life for everybody. And this is unlimited. Whatever life is given to you by the pranic energy is unlimited.

It is not necessary that you will die and you will be forgotten. There are human examples to show us. Guru Nanak came in the physical body, lived, talked, preached, helped others, elevated everybody. Then he was ever with us, now he is with ever us. Nobody forgot him when he was alive. Nobody forgets him now.

In the Sikh way of life, there is no secret.

---

[38] *Pranic shakti:* the creativity and power given to the being through the breath.

ਆਪਿ ਜਪੈ ਅਵਰਹ ਨਾਮੁ ਜਪਾਵੈ ਵਡ ਸਮਰਥ ਤਾਰਨ ਤਰਨ ॥੧॥

Aap japai avrah naam japaavai vad samrath taaran taran.

It's a very simple thing for prosperity, for purpose, and for projection of life:
meditate on God and inspire others to meditate.

— Guru Arjan Dev ji, *Siri Guru Granth Sahib*, page 1206, line 9, as translated by Yogi Bhajan

The mind is always there to remind us that there are weaknesses, that there are handicaps and that we are handicapped by many things. Yet, this covers all weaknesses.

With simplicity, we can become very wise. Look at the diet of the Sikhs in the early times. It was the very best diet—very simple. And they were so healthy. Their bodies were well built and they were always there to serve. With service, they earned friendship forever, from everybody. It wasn't that A is my friend and B is my enemy and C is my acquaintance and D is just someone I know. No, they served everyone. Whenever a call came, when a need came, they came out and they were with people. They were dependable people, serviceful people, projective people—people with smiles and glowing faces.

The *Shabad Guru* of *Siri Guru Granth* is going to prevail, and the quantum impact of the sound and *naad* is going to be very effective for the human. Understand that in the first half of the 21st century, our entire knowledge is going to be absolutely obsolete. The computer will use a chip. The chip will have memory, and the memory will be in the millions. It can go up to four billion. Can you believe a little chip can retain four billion memorable thoughts? And then what will happen is that the human will have to have a power to match up with that, even if we are unable to cope with the work. We always say there are fewer hours and more work. That's a common feeling we have.

But actually what is going to happen is that there's going to be so much information, so much knowledge available that what they say is, every illiterate person will become absolutely wise and every wise person will become insane. That's how much knowledge there will be. So how will you retain the balance? How will you cover the distance? How will you relax in life? That is where sophistication will come in. That is where the *Shabad Guru* will come in.

An intermediary will not be needed. A person will read the permutation and combination of the *sutras*[39] in the *Siri Guru Granth Sahib*. He will go through it and in other languages he will understand the meaning of what the *Guru* is saying. When the understanding is inside, when the words are in the heart of a person, then that person will be very, very balanced. Extremely balanced. Highly sophisticated and absolutely balanced. What a wonderful world that will be.

You know, you can be very rich and not balanced. You can be very poor and not balanced. You can be very macho and not balanced. The beauty of a human is to just be a human. And a balanced human is so powerful. First of all, it gives a satisfaction to the person

---

[39] *Sutras:* couplets or verses.

who is enjoying it. You know how beautiful it is to be human? We are human first. Then after that we are Sikhs of the *Guru*, and the word of the *Guru* is in our heart and our understanding is in our head. The words of the *Guru* say these things to us and we follow them.

It's a strange thing. Just watch what I'm saying, "I follow myself because I have the *Guru's* words in me. The *Guru's* word in me I follow. Therefore, I follow myself." Look how sovereign we are, how free we are, how clear our consciousness is. We are not subject to anybody. "I understand." There's not a fear. There's a vastness. There's a joy to serve and hug everybody and tell everybody how great the universe is. And the attitude of gratitude builds confidence in other people. Then the relationships are very beautiful.

The power of lust and the luster of the moment is not what a human can continue to create. After a while the nervous system will fall apart. You are not together. But to get together and to be together, one has to go in-depth into the *Siri Guru Granth*—the word, the meaning and the purpose.

We say *Wahe Guru*. What a vastness we believe in. *Wahe*, all that there is is because of the *Guru*. All that is *gur prasaad*[40]. All that is because of the wisdom of the *Guru*. You see what freedom there is in that? "It's not me. It's something higher, bigger and better than me. I have found my best, I have found my vastness. That's my *Guru*."

And that is what *Guru* means to a Sikh. What *Shabad Guru* means to a Sikh. It's not that there is another body you have to carry on your shoulder. No. It is the wisdom, it is the Word, it is that sophisticated correction and guidance that is in my heart, that I follow. I am enriched by it and I go by it, step by step.

There are a lot of things coming at us. When there's light, a lot of moths come. A lot of tests come. A lot of tragedies come. A lot of challenges come. Every challenge has to be met. Because that is graduation—the test of a human identity, human endurance, human faith and human beauty. You cannot NOT have tests and challenges in life. Otherwise life would become very boring and then you would have no juice in it.

That's the life of a Sikh. He relates to the entire universe, and relates to everyone around him. Inside he's so enriched—enriched by the energy of the *Shabad Guru*. He knows,

ਏ ਮਨ ਮੇਰਿਆ ਤੂ ਸਦਾ ਰਹੁ ਹਰਿ ਨਾਲੇ ॥

Ay man mayri-aa too sadaa rahu har naalay.

Oh my mind, be with God all the time.

— Guru Amar Das, *Anand Sahib*, Pauree 2, as translated by Yogi Bhajan

So he is reminded and he remembers. He feels and he understands. And he is that way. When he is talking, walking or dealing with somebody, he feels God within. He feels the wisdom of the *Guru* within. So basically there is no karma. That's the way this *dharma* is and that's the way this *dharma* augments life.

---

[40] *Gur prasaad:* Gift or blessing of the **Guru.**

You who are walking on this path of the *Guru* have to understand it that way. Don't measure things by money, by *maya*. Gain and loss, achievement, have and have-nots—that is by the will of God. It is His universe. It's not mine. It's not yours, but sometimes you do not understand. You think this world is "mine."

We are all takers. We take. We take from one God. If we can all feel that we take from one God, then we'll never fight amongst ourselves. Sometimes, you see a child. A child grabs something from another child. The mother comes and she says, "Don't worry. I'll give you more." And that is how God is.

ਉਸ ਤੇ ਚਉਗੁਨ ਕਰੈ ਨਿਹਾਲੁ ॥

Us tay cha-ugun karai nihaal.

Sometimes He gives you four times.

— Guru Arjan Dev ji, *Siri Guru Granth Sahib*, page 268, line 11, as translated by Yogi Bhajan

Then what do you have?

This is a fantastic way of life. When we speak *Guru's* words with our tongue, we are purified.

CHAPTER TEN

UNDERSTAND YOUR PSYCHE

As we grow older, we feel more fatigue. We do not admit it, but we all mentally become insensitive. Instead of living on our normal intuition, we start living by our ego. Psychologically and biologically, the ego is meant to sustain our identity. But ego is not the purpose of our life.

There are two types of people: those who live odd and indifferently and those who live even and happily. There is a human need to reflect your identity. You will reflect your identity so that you can affect the identity. That's how we mutually talk to each other. We are social. Sometimes in that reflection, our psyches get entangled and we are deeply in love. When we cannot follow the rhythm of our own psyche, we deflect ourselves and we lose the relationship.

You do fashion. You look in the mirror and try to look pretty. You may end up looking ugly, but—according to your ego—you have to look pretty. According to your spirit you may be very ugly. You talk too much because you want to convince people you are good.

Well, if you are good, you are good. Why do you have to talk about it? What's the reason that you want to convince other people and gain their friendship? Why do you want friends? Because you are alone? Because you are not sure that this whole universe is in friendship with you? If you tune into the inter-related psyche of the universe, you don't need relatives, you don't need friends, you don't need to ask for anything. If you don't believe this statement, look at the children. They get everything. They can make a mess out of you if they want. They start crying in the middle of something and they can disturb the entire audience, and you have nothing against them.

Yet, if you just make one wrong move as an adult, any person will tell you to shut up. Do you understand, as we grow in life, how much impact we lose? For children, food is free, bathing is free, jogging and walking are free, the mother is a nurse, and the father is a guardian. Where are those facilities now? You get up in the morning, go to work, come back in the evening, exercise. You're afraid to grow old, afraid to grow lonely. You're trying to correct your relationships.

The child is there and everybody relates to the child—not to the relatives or the friends or the parents. Everybody relates to the child. And you? Nobody relates to you. So it is called "psychosomatic inter-jamming of the psyche." In simple English, in psychology, it is called "social sickness." All of you are fatigued by social sickness. The pressure of society takes a very heavy toll. Ultimately, that toll slows you down with a powerful insensitivity. You try to take shelter under religion, social groups, social ideas, and other good charitable work. When you are young, you take drugs, drink, dance, eat and party.

Recently, somebody was in a lot of trouble. The person asked me for help. I understood his psychology, psychiatry and medical background and I said, "I can't help you. You have gone too far."

He said, "No, honest to God, I want to be helped. I don't want to live like this. I feel I give people a lot of pain. I am very antisocial. I am very reserved and I doubt everything in life. I am miserable. Everybody is miserable. I don't want this life."

I said, "Look, son, if you doubt yourself, you will fall into the pit of doubts and you will never make sense. If you act and react, you go forward and go backwards—it's not very healthy, either. If you answer the call of *dharma*, and if you have no heart in it, you won't make any sense."

"What should I do?"

"Do what is required. You need higher energy. You need your higher psyche. You should purify you so you can enjoy life."

"What should I do?"

"Give me my fee."

He said, "I will give you anything you want."

I said, "Not that way. Lay it out. Put some money here. Let me see how much you want to pay for this counsel."

"Fifty dollars?"

"No, a little more."

"Seventy-five? A hundred? A hundred and eight?"

I said, "You are very chronically stupid. You want to get wisdom for a hundred and eight bucks? See? You have started wrong."

"What should I have done?"

"You should have said, 'In God's name, in *Guru's* name, give me your advice.' Then, there would have been no choice. I wanted to test how you measure things in life. You measure things in money. Correct your manners. But you can't correct them. It is in you. Like a cavity is in a tooth. Like pain is in the nerve. You can't help it."

"What should I do?"

I said, "For thirty-one minutes a day, do the one-minute breath meditation."

This is a story of a man who is grateful today, who is successful today, who has become compassionate. He has realized himself. Why? It's so simple. You live the by breath. You die by the breath. If you meditate on your breath, the *Pavan Guru*, the knowledge of the *pranic vidya* of creation and creativity and all incarnations, will dawn on you. Some may take a little time. Some may take a long time. But the path is the same. The procedure is the same. You will start winning yourself. You will start valuing your breath. You will start valuing your environments. You will start valuing your projections and one day you will be surprised. Everyone, in turn, will value you.

If you watch the development of a human from an impersonal camera, you will find him very afraid and scared. He is an extremely lonely person. Everything that he does on the surface is to get rid of that fear, that loneliness. People can't even sleep. You have dreams. Dreams.

Once, just for fun, I started looking at somebody's palm. Twenty people wanted to get their palms read. Isn't it amazing? You all want to know your tomorrow, but you don't care to know your today. We call ourselves civilized human beings with churches, synagogues, temples, religious teachers, yoga, swamis, preachers, psychologists, sociological workers and counselors with tons of status. Yet, you are all mentally alone. Fifteen thousand books a year get published—fiction, nonfiction, drama, biographies, tons of magazines, libraries, radio, television—but you are unfortunate and still alone. You have never been taught how to turn this loneliness into power. You don't have a practice. Therefore, everyday you become harsher and harsher and harder and harder. You have never been taught to become you. You have been taught to become "somebody."

All these years we have been taught wrong because we have never been taught to be peaceful. We have never been taught how to achieve peace of mind when everything is upside down. Our existence is not a peaceful, tranquil existence.

Therefore life has one simple challenge: act—don't react. Calm yourself and claim yourself. When you hold up a torch, it takes away the darkness for a long distance. When you reflect, your psyche takes away indifference.

Once in a court there were two attorneys giving their arguments. One said, "The guy is innocent." The other said "No. He is a criminal." They argued to the jury. They argued to the judge. They argued to the audience.

The jury said in its decision, "Though there is a lot of evidence to prove the man guilty, we say he is innocent." It created a big uproar.

So later on, when they could get a chance, they asked the jurors, "How did you come to this decision? When there is over sixty percent evidence against him, how can you say the guy is innocent?"

One of the jurors said, "You want to know how? Throughout the proceedings, he was a very calm, quiet and most peaceful person. Isn't that his nature?"

They said, "Yes but you know this . . ."

The juror said, "What do you mean 'this …'? Prove that in his life he is violent. In our hearts, we have searched through the evidence. The evidence that comes from the government is government evidence, but all the civil evidence that came on his side said only one thing: he is a gentleman. He is a peaceful man. He is a very sweet man. And how he has been involved in this, we can't say."

You do not know that when you speak for yourself or when somebody speaks for you, there is somebody else who will also speak for you, and that is your character and projection. That is your self. Your self is the strongest thing you have.

We have a very powerful magnetic psyche. We can just attract things. We can get things. But do we have that training? No. We sweat, hassle and go after things. Is that living? Hustlers? Poachers? Going after things? Beggars? Seeking protection from the powerful to the weak? Your own dog will not do it. He has a master and the rest of the world has nothing to do with that dog. You have a God. And you are beggars? Hustlers? Requesting everything. Everything is "Please, can I, may I, should I?" Would you love me? Would you like me? What kind of life is this? Is it life?

When I first came to Canada from India, the circumstances became totally desperate. All that was there, was taken away—whooosh. That's what happened to me. I came with a perfect macho image. And it happened. Whooosh. Everything was gone. I said to myself, "There is a purpose. There is a mutual purpose to this challenge. There is a mutual purpose for this pain." It was so insane. I didn't have a coat or a sweater. The temperature was minus forty-five degrees outside. The wind was blowing at sixty miles an hour and was about three feet of snow on the ground. Every day it was snowing. It tended my heart.

I saw somebody on Church Street lying down on a bench. He started talking to me. And he got up and said, "Hey holy man."

I said, "How do you know I am holy?"

"Nobody can walk in this winter other than me and you."

"What are you doing here?"

"Drinking. I am in ecstasy. I am warm. You are in ecstasy. You are warm. You are warm hearted."

"How do you know all this?"

"You mean anyone born of a woman can stand here and talk to me in this cold? And you have only one cotton shirt on you?"

"Well it's an obligation. You got up and you wanted to talk to me. So I am talking to you."

He said, "Do me a favor. I want real liquor. Real."

"Okay I will send it to you."

"I'll wait."

I came to the house of yoga and I said to one student, "There is a drunkard bum, he wants real liquor. Can you oblige him?"

The student said, "Thank you sir. I'll just go."

THE 26 STEPS OF WISDOM

The head is dead without the spine, and the twenty-six vertebrae are the twenty-six steps of wisdom. There are twenty-six parts in the skull—if they are not adjusted with a turban you are dull. There are twenty-six bones in your foot that have to be adjusted right—without that adjustment you can never be bright.

1. Those who do not move, move the Universe. Those who move, don't move anything.
2. Feelings and emotions are like waves on oceans—no depth. Without depth there are no oceans and no waves. Then you are living notions.
3. Those who have to lead must be like a star with an altitude and attitude of perfection.
4. God is single but all prevailing.
5. Work speaks for itself.
6. Wisdom, character and consciousness conquer everything.
7. Count your blessings and save yourself from the tyranny of time and space.
8. Be kind, conscious and compassionate. The whole world will be your friend.
9. There is nothing naked in the nature. Even trees have bark.
10. Going without knowing is a social suicide.
11. Don't forget God because God doesn't forget anything.
12. All those men who create their own castles, God creates for them equal hassles.
13. I, I, I. You will never open your Third Eye.
14. Ego is a bubble that creates nothing but trouble.
15. Face and grace can win every race.
16. There is no match to character. All characteristics of the Universe will fit in.
17. The best desire is to be desireless.
18. The best anger is to be angry at your faults.
19. The best attachment is to be gracefully excellent and gratefully compassionate.
20. The best attachment is to be attached to your character and consciousness — and prove it through your intelligence.
21. The best love is to serve all equally.
22. The best pride is to pray for everyone.
23. The best greed is to agree to be the forklift of every existence.
24. The best lust is to lure yourself to be graceful.
25. To be great is to be great and full.
26. Tomorrow always becomes today and yesterday is always gone. Therefore, life is a gift. Don't drift or create a rift. Be happy so long as the breath is on.

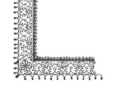

So he went. The student brought a bottle of something and he went there. But there was nobody. He had gone. He was not there. I saw the student coming back and I said, "What happened? The bottle is in your hand. You didn't give it to him?"

He said, "There is nobody there. He is gone."

"Okay. Then you take it to your home. Somebody will drink it who believes in drinking. You Canadians all drink like fish."

"We are vegetarian. We don't drink."

"Give it to somebody."

I came back from the yoga house and there was a shopkeeper, a general shopkeeper. I will never forget his grace and his greatness. He called me and took me into the shop and I said, "How come you are so kind to me?"

He said, "This is a bundle that I have tied up. I know you won't take it for free, so give me two dollars."

I said, "What is this bundle? I never asked you for anything."

"No. You curse me everyday."

"Man, I don't curse you. What do I curse you for?"

"I have this shop on one block. I sell all kind of clothes and you walk almost naked through the street in the freezing snow."

"Well, everything of mine was lost."

"No. I am not giving it to you. Give me two dollars."

I gave him two dollars and I started checking the bundle. There was one small Minolta camera, a spy camera. I said, "How did you know about this?"

He said, "Weren't you working in intelligence? I just put it in if you want to have some photos." I couldn't believe it.

Well, I took that coat and put it on me and I brought those warm clothes home. I tried my best not to weep for a couple of hours but the tears started flowing from my eyes like rain. For the first time as a human I understood—God takes care of things. He understands people. All of a sudden, it came to me,

ਸੈਲ ਪਥਰ ਮਹਿ ਜੰਤ ਉਪਾਏ ਤਾ ਕਾ ਰਿਜਕੁ ਆਗੈ ਕਰਿ ਧਰਿਆ ॥ ਮੇਰੇ ਮਾਧਉ ਜੀ ਸਤਸੰਗਤਿ ਮਿਲੇ ਸੁ ਤਰਿਆ ॥

Sail pat'har meh jant upaa-ay taa kaa rijak aagai kar dhari-aa.
Mayray maadhau jee sat sangat milay so tariaa.

God provides the provision to even those creatures that He has created in the stone. The livelihood for what He has created in the stones He has already placed there. My great lord, in the congregation one goes across all difficulties.

— Guru Arjan, *Rehiraas Sahib*, as translated by Yogi Bhajan

What do we have here? We have a sense of congregation, a sense of consolidation, a sense of sharing. What is this lecture? It is just a cause. This is our psyche, the flow of our identity for each other, for our understanding. It's our meditation when we get ready and come here to sit, sing for a while, listen to a talk, try to ponder over things. But while we do that, we exchange the psyche. That enrichment happens. Those thirty trillion cells and their most booming power intermixes and creates a sense of purity, of piety. *Sat sangat milay so tariaa*: The purpose of this congregation is so that we can elevate ourselves.

I travel everywhere. I don't have to search like lord Buddha all my life to find out why we are suffering. We are suffering because we do not trust ourselves. It's that simple. I see this common disease, this sickness: there is no self trust.

We look in the mirror, and we want to look good. Or we take notes, and then make speeches. We want to convince each other. Look at how emotional we are. We shake hands and say, "Come on. Cheer up. How are you?"

What's the need of this? Don't we know each other? Love each other? There is no reason for me to tell you I love you and there is no reason for you to tell me you love me. But there is a common reason—the only reason that we coexist at this time and space. And it's a gift. Why drift from that gift? Why do you care that somebody is fat, small, or skinny? Why do dimensions bother you? Why does intelligence bother you? Are you not intelligent enough to understand that this is the time we are together? It's very important. And it's very important that, at this time, you are just you. Whether you are sick, unhealthy, hungry, tired—you are you. Just that. That's very important. When you are not you, understand how miserable that situation is.

Within a relationship, there are two individual identities. Male and a female, male and a male, female and female. Child and parents, parents and child. Whatever you want to identify it as. But the net result is that it has to be decided on values. If a woman wants what she wants and it is without values, she is actually going to self-destruct. If a male wants what he wants and it has no positive values, then it is not going to work it out. If commotions can make emotions, and if our feelings are all healing, we would be living in the heavens.

Let's break this deadly, monotonous, low, social fear and open up this congested brain.

We should work the third neurological plate, which sets our pattern, our personality and our projection. There is a part in our brain called the third neurological plate cycle. It is in the hemispheres of the brain and it sets the pattern of our personality. What I am telling you about today, they will find out medically in a hundred years. Let them research it. There is a little stem of the brain. It has three rings that set your temperament, your metabolism and your pattern. Additionally, the effectiveness of your personality is in how you speak. When you get up in the morning and open your eyes to be yourself, that first minute sets the whole frequency of the day. If one day, you get up and feel indifferent to yourself for that first minute, then during the whole day, everything will be indifferent to you. There is nothing wrong within you, but the frequency of your psyche and the frequency of the psyche of the day will not connect.

There are two parts of your body that are undeveloped: the upper palate in the mouth and the frontal lobe. The upper palate has eighty-four meridian points. The thalamus and the hypothalamus are on top of it. That controls your personality in terms of your automatic habits. And that can be organized, developed and set.

The frontal lobe is where your personality is manufactured every day for day-to-day work. The total personality comes out of it. It is where your systematic work or your expertise is expressed. It's through the development of the frontal lobe that a doctor becomes a specialist, an engineer becomes a professor and a human becomes a saint.

> There are two ways of living: one way is to go after things, the other is to sit and be and let it come to you. You can choose which way you want to live.

You don't become a saint by being born in the house of a saint. You don't become a doctor by being born in a house of a doctor. You have to learn, then become learned, experienced and candid. You have to show the steadfastness of your expertise. Then people will trust you. Then you don't need fantasy, and you don't need to hassle. Things will come to you wherever you are.

There are two ways of living: one way is to go after things, the other is to sit and be and let it come to you. You can choose which way you want to live.

Every person has the right of progression and every progressive self has to have a definite discipline so that he or she can create a frequency and a projection. To us that is God. If we are energetic, vibrant, unafraid, relaxed and happy, that is God. The opposite of that is the devil. But we know how to create God, so why talk of the devil?

Because the power is inside us. We have to work with our own neurological system. Meditation is for nothing else but to set up the neurological balance. It's very incorrectly taught in the west. They think meditation means something. It's nothing. It's simply to set up the glandular and neurological balance.

The time has come. Become your own master. Stop chasing masters. Become your own reality. Stop chasing religion. Become your own God. Stop chasing God. Be you. In the beginning, in the middle, in the end, it is you and you alone. Live well in your inner peace, in your inner strength and when you feel weak, call on your soul, your friend. It costs much less than a telephone call.

On average, you breathe fifteen times a minute. Suppose you have to live one hundred years. If you breathe one breath a minute, you can live fifteen hundred years. Because life is measured by the breath, not by the years or the calendars. If you sit down and breathe one breath a minute, in exactly thirty seconds, you will find you are talking to yourself. In three minutes you can get over any kind of mood that a psychiatrist cannot get you out of for centuries. Why are you suffering?

This is how I describe it scientifically. The macro- and microwave continuity of the psyche of projection will always interfere with the totality of the whole universe. Where the individual is bombarded with the mega million thoughts and variations of other people, and those variations create brain earthquakes. But if a person is a practitioner of certain scientific knowledge in which he or she can balance him or herself, then the balanced situation can take all those attacks and normalize them to remain as an individual. Under those circumstances you will be under your personal self. You will be your own personal managers and you will be personally happy persons, because then you will know the self.

There is a story about a young man who was walking who saw a lion coming. The lion started running after him. There was an old man who said, "Oh young man, don't run. Go up the tree." The man immediately grabbed the tree, went up and sat there. The lion tried to get him, but eventually got tired and went away. The young man came down and said to the old man, "I want to thank you."

The old man said, "Learn in the future my son. When calamity hits you, elevate yourself." He said, "You are a young, inexperienced guy. You wanted to run away from the lion. The lion would have gotten you. But when you elevated yourself, he had no way to catch you."

In every thought in our life, we must elevate. If we know meditation, if we know concentration, if we know anything in our life, we should learn one thing: elevate.

You know, there are religions like Judaism, Islam, Hinduism, Buddhism and all that kind of thing. They are only one word: Jehovah, Hallelujah, Rama and Sata Nama. If you just understand the first syllable, every religion has one word. That's it. And then they make a big philosophy out of it. Actually it is one word. "God." If you meet a Jew, he will say Jehovah. If you meet a Christian, he will say hallelujah. If you meet a Hindu, he is going to say Rama. If you meet a Muslim, he is going to say La-Illah and if you meet a Sikh, he is going to say Sata Nama. Actually it is one word. They don't have more than one word. The rest is to collect money.

I used to go to all the countries and meet all the religious leaders because I am the head of a religion, myself, so it was very possible. They would come to have a cup of tea, and for one year, I would ask everybody this same question: "Why are we different?" And the answer that came was, "Turf." I couldn't understand what "turf" meant. It means the collection basket, the money, the political influence, the congregation. That's all.

Everybody is afraid that I will steal their students. I have more students than I can handle. They are already a headache. God, these people should take some of my students—they are not easy kids. But these religious people are always afraid. They judge a spiritual person by how many students he has. How many ashrams he has. How much political influence he has. They don't judge him by how content, contained and wise he is. How peaceful, neutral and impersonal he is. And how strong he is to crack open your head and put a new brain in it. Because you have never met a teacher.

There is one description about what happens when you meet your teacher. The description is from Ramanand Paramahansa. He said, "Before I met my teacher, I was very wise, very clean, very clear, well respected and well acknowledged. The moment I met my teacher, I became nothing. It was a very bad omen. But later on I realized, I had become wealthy."

In the West, you have not met teachers because teachers come here to depend on you and you are catered to—because you are all window-shoppers. One day, you will become real students and you shall become real masters. If a seed does not go into the dust, and if it does not split, it never sprouts. It can never become a tree again and it cannot give more seeds.

The time has come. You have to be you. Neither very haughty nor second-hand fashion. Be a beautiful, bountiful and blissful human. Nobody can create you. God created you in His own image. Don't create your own images. There is just one image of you—as you being the being of God. It's very human and that is what the Age of Aquarius is all about. It will be an age of humans and peace, love and service and we shall all be relatives. The small wars and fights will go. Humanity will prevail again. As the Berlin wall fell, other walls will fall. We will all be united under one God. One Spirit. One Self.

If you can keep on practicing what you have learned, it will keep you healthy, happy and holy. You have nine holes. Watch what comes in and goes out of those holes. That will make you holy. You have nine holes and two hands and two legs. That's called thirteen. You are born with thirteen, you will live with thirteen, and you will die with thirteen. Whosoever controls all thirteen will live forever in peace and prosperity.

I have a dream that one day you will grow and carry this *dharma* to serve humanity. It will be very easy on you if you leave behind your shortcomings, forget about your miseries and just serve and uplift others in the name of the Lord. Whatever religion you were or you are or you will be, uplift people and reach out.

Chapter Eleven

Ten Sacred Secrets
of Success

Life is not a moment or a mood. Life is forever. We want to understand the main fears that nobody wants to talk about. They are there. Regardless of whether you like it or not, you shall face them one day in one situation or another.

The question arises because we have these ten problems hidden within us. They come one after the other. First of all, we don't want to face them. Secondly, we avoid them. And then we get stuck in a ditch. It is very simple. Because, a) there is a problem, b) there is a solution, c) there is a result of the effort.

Life is not meant for you to just be a joker or a yo-yo. Life is to for you to face. The bigger the challenge, the better the conviction, the best the results. Nobody is above challenge. Life is a challenge. Whenever time and space meet, a cause will happen. A cause will have an effect. And you have got to face it. That's why I say to you that your happiness is in you. It cannot be in anybody else. Have a clean state of mind and meditate. Clean your thoughts yourself and don't lay them on others.

THE TEN SACRED SECRETS OF SUCCESS

1. **Learning Is not a Weakness**

    Time and space and breath of life is the living trinity of life. Every process is a moment; every moment is a process. Learning is to gain wisdom. It gives a grip on our discipline and disciple becomes the Master. Master creates the legacy; legacy lives forever; mortal becomes Immortal.
    Oh Yogi, life is a living chance forever …

2. **If Somebody Is Avoiding Reaching Out to You, You Reach Out (Knowing is the Knowledge)**

    If the head has gone cold, the heart has gone frozen; if hatred in somebody has eaten up the heat of life and there is no warmth coming to you, but still the body is vibrating and the breath of life is keeping it warm—reach out and melt away all the coldness through your humor and boldness. So that the flower of friendship can blossom and you can enjoy the fragrance.
    Oh Yogi, this is knowingness …

3. **Be the Altar—not the Alternative**

    Between time and space there is a place that is the altar of human legacy. Each individual must identify this altar and worship it. It will give personality, purpose and prosperity. Any alternative to this is to lose the gratefulness, the grace and the glow of life.
    Oh Yogi, this is the sacred secret of prosperity …

4. **Let Your Manners Speak for You, Let Your Deeds Prove You and Let Your Deliverance Impress You**

    Everyone has a mission. Every mission has a magnitude. To fulfill and deliver the essence of magnitude, one requires manner and attitude. When one does it with devotion and conviction, success comes from all sides.
    Oh Yogi, this is the sacred secret of success …

5. **Work Never Waits—Those Who Wait Have not Started Yet**

    Nobody can stop the time. Time creates the space. We move between longitude and latitude. It is the attitude that works out and completes every work for us.
    Oh Yogi, this is the sacred secret of deliverance …

6. **Excuses, Avoidance, and Delays Will not Stop the Consequences**

    Every sequence will have consequences. Every action will have reaction. Every start will have finish. Every beginning will have end. Our insecurity

delays our achievement. Our excuses show our weakness, and our delay lays the foundation of frustration. The Perfect One, God Almighty, made us perfect to face every challenge and be a victor. As every artist wants to see his art the best, so our divinity wants us to conquer our duality.
Oh Yogi, this is the sacred secret of victory …

7. **Pros and Cons: Check Properly—It will Save You from Con Games**
Play no games. Get straight to the strategy and establish the state and status with your statesmanship. Reach out to everyone with a diplomatic art and loving communication.
Oh Yogi, this is the sacred secret of winning friends …

8. **Be a Statesman and a Diplomat**
If you have a longing to belong, love and reverence are your handy tools to build a leadership to sail through the stormy ocean, and you enter the port of peace and tranquility.
Oh Yogi, this is the sacred secret of leadership …

9. **Your Individuality, Your Attire and Your Attitude—**
That Counts above All
You must have vitality to create virtues. You must have values to honor virtues. Your honorable performance will give people trust. Your reverence and love give people belief in you and your honesty and character will give people faith in you.
Oh Yogi, this is the sacred secret of creating lasting memory of self or memorial in the heart of others …

10. **Act Three Ways—Action, Support, Cover**
(Must Include Safe Place for Retreat)
Every action has a reaction that is equal and opposite. What comes, goes. What is born must die. But the wisdom is to create a legacy that is perpetual, everlasting guidance for all. Every action force in a strategy must have a cover force and a support force and a place of retreat to take care of the casualties. With that planning, one can reach fulfillment.
Oh Yogi, this is the sacred secret of joy and happiness in life …

Blessed is Guru Nanak, the great source of wisdom.
Blessed is Guru Gobind Singh, the great example of courage.
Blessed is Guru Ram Das, the great lord of miracles.
And blessed is the *Khalsa Panth*, the great avenue of purity, piety and power.
Blessed are all, Oh Yogi, who follow this path of wisdom …

That's why there are problems. People like to talk to each other. People like to lean on each other. People like to offend each other. These are people who don't meditate. A man who meditates doesn't need anybody. He doesn't even need God. I have seen people in my life who, when you tell them about God, say, "What?" Because they don't feel that God is a foreign identity. They feel what we say. "*Hamee ham braham ham*. We are the we, and we are the God." Their tranquility and their explanation are so unique and so vast, so calm and quiet.

In anger, a person acts like a tyrant. But given just the very appearance of calmness and quietness in the body language, and the psyche calms people down.

For any person who is shakable, a challenge is something to be drunk right there and then like a milkshake. Then what's left? An empty glass. Take challenges as normal. Face them with sweetness and deliver them with perfection. The victory shall be yours.

People like to lean on each other. They want to present a picture. They want to spread their fear. There will always be fear. No matter how secure you are, you will be afraid. Because there are two forces that move you: one is love; the other is fear. There is no other force for living.

Love is such a beautiful mirage. Love neither buys the groceries nor does it pay the bills. But it's such a wanting pull. Make an appointment with your beloved at 6:00 p.m. If there is hell and heaven, a traffic jam on earth, if the police stop everything—you will sneak through. You will be there. It's the attractive force. Logic and reason stop when there is love. Questions and answers are gone. Insecurity and security do not exist.

It is just that moment. It doesn't matter if you are even in love with your dog. One day I saw somebody in love with his dog, driving a hundred and twenty miles an hour to be there to feed the dog at four o'clock. Can you believe it? The guy had an accident. He was in a hospital. All he asked the doctor was, "Is my dog fed?"

Three days later he woke up. The first question he asked was, "Is my dog okay?"

What can you do with this guy? His dog caused his accident and totaled the car. There were about forty or fifty stitches all over his body. Just imagine it. He was driving a hundred and twenty miles an hour. Thank God he had his seat belt on. The whole thing was a mess because he was running late. As if it's a crucial hour. As if the dog will never eat after four o'clock. What an appointment. Can you believe it? That's the craziness.

Fear is a constant, consistent companion. You are all afraid. Therefore you work. Mostly you don't work from love. You work from fear and your need for security, competition and jealousy. The industry of the whole world is based on your fear that you are handicapped.

You are miserable and you are an idiot. How much more of an idiot can you be? You don't trust yourself. You don't know whether you are beautiful or not. You don't know whether you are wise or not. Your wisdom is a comparative study. Your happiness is a comparative study. Your life is a comparative study. If you really want to look at it, whenever you compare, you are not sure. So you are not sure whether you are an idiot or not. That's the first sign of an idiot—that the person is never sure. Do you understand how poor you all are? Because you are never sure you are rich. It's so funny.

If you are perfect, you are ten percent. If all the environments and good luck are with you, that is another ten percent. Eighty percent is still unknown. So who is talking to who?

The idea is to learn and acknowledge that eighty percent is unknown and intuitively follow what the eighty percent is. Twenty percent can go on commission. You are banging along based on your twenty percent. Twenty percent doesn't mean a thing. Eighty percent is always unknown.

If you sincerely look at your life, you will find a surprising thing. You never expected the good, nor did you expect the bad. You are amazed at the miracles. So every life is full of miracles.

In this human body—as you are—the destiny is set. But the fate is always competing with it. The fight is between those two—not you. You are the puppet. But if your mind is clear, the destiny and the distance will be done perfectly. If the mind is not clear, if it's not with you, if it's clogged up, then fate will take over and rub your nose in the dirt. There is nothing to it.

We are all one mala—one rosary—linked with one thread, the breath of life.

All the men and women, who have tried to succeed in their lives, have lost the game in the hands of their own insecurity—in the hands of their own fear.

Nobody believes it but this entire universe is just one person. There are no two people. There is one link of the breath of life that comes from me to you, to you, to you, to you, to you, to you. It's all linked with one thread. When it gets disconnected, you are gone. We are all one mala—one rosary—linked with one thread of the breath of life. And the realm of our id is only two seconds, on average.

Nobody is above anybody. Nobody is below anybody. We make it so. And when we put people above us, we have to carry that weight. When we put them down below us, we have to drag them. And we get tired. What kind of life is that?

So my idea is, please realize, that you are the most perfect that the Perfect could ever create. There is no ugliness in you. If you don't believe me, when you were a little child, you were loved exactly by all. Since you have grown up, many people hate you. Many people love you.

When I was a little boy, nobody ever hated me. But now, nobody even has the right to love me. They don't know what to do with me. Right now, I am sixty-two years old, and I say, "Come on, love me."

It's not practical. How can you love me? I already know you. Love is an intoxication. It's a goof. It's a mirage. It is a romance. Romance is a mirage by thoughts, and love is a mirage by faith. Do you know what love is? You believe so. You want so. You are so. Actually what it is—is nothing. You don't want to look at it. And romance is thoughts and thoughts and thoughts and thoughts. But you know, "All is one and one is all." What is there to love? What is there to romance? What is there to hate? What is there to put down? Put up?

You all want to be beautiful, right? All of you are ugly. Because you don't trust that you are beautiful. Try to be beautiful. Everybody is putting out an effort to be successful, to be beautiful, to be rich, to be something. Sometimes I wonder, will these people ever have time for themselves? Just to be? Just to be to be? "*Hamee ham braham ham*. We are the we and we are the God?"

Those who believe in Nanak, his first line says it, "*Ek Ong Kaar*. There is one God. Every creature is His creation." That's it. Full stop. Doesn't go anywhere. That's the beginning, that's the middle and that's the end.

Somebody was telling me today about something that I should have. I winked and I said, "It's not meant to be."

Because how can a thing come to you that has an inferior aura, even though it has a wonderful mark on it? Every material object has a foot-and-a-half aura. Every living animal—even the birds—has a three-and-a-half-foot aura. Every human may have up to a nine-foot aura. If the auras are not creating that attractive mechanism, and if the magnet is not strong, they are not going to join. And it must create an opposite polarity to come together. If the polarity is the same, they will repel each other.

An idiot will love a wise person; a wise person will love an idiot. A wise person will never love a wise person. They will conflict to death. Ugly wants the beauty, beauty wants the ugly. If you have two beautiful things, what are you going to get out of that? Equals never meet. Parallels never meet. Opposites do. But you don't want opposition. What a boring life you want to live. Create opposition if it is not there. Learn one thing from me—I create it.

If somebody says, "I love you," I say, "Love me more."

They don't know what to do. All they say is, "He is not satisfied." Well, fine, I am not satisfied. Why should I be satisfied? Satisfaction is boredom. Who wants to be satisfied? What is satisfaction? Nothing. It's pure boredom.

"I have achieved God."

Big deal! Then what? What next? I still have to breathe. I still have to go to the bathroom. I still have to wear clothes. What's the idea of meeting God? I met Him yesterday. What happened today? The work was the same. Every report got signed, every check was recorded and every telephone call was made. The class had to be taught. Big deal!

Once you are acknowledged as a status, it's boredom. Every day you tell a king to "Get ready and sit on the throne," he itches.

You know the job of a judge? He presides. Everybody rises up. So-and-so is coming. He sits down. Everybody sits down and then he starts. Can you believe from nine to five he sits on a chair and can't move? Have you seen them? He sits and sits and sits and sits and the drama goes on. Isn't it boring?

Once I was security officer. They told me that for my next promotion I would have to become an income tax officer. But I reverted back to the customs office. They said, "Why? It's a promotion."

I said, "Sitting on a chair the whole day and passing wind? Forget it. I am not going to do it. A six-by-six room? As a customs officer, my jurisdiction starts from here—fifteen hundred miles and goes that way for fifteen hundred miles. What the hell is going to tie me to that room? These rooms I assign to other people."

That is no life. Life is fun when you sit in a ditch, put on a wireless, and pass the message. Or ask the accountants, "Has the check gone yet or not?"

That's fun. But is it fun to sit in an office and do the same thing every morning, afternoon and evening? That's not life. But some people, if you ask them to move, they can't. You develop your psyche by your fears. Your fears are what limit you. Your fears cut you off from the totality of life.

The core of us is like the earth's core—it has nothing but molten lava. That's all it is.

The molten lava creates the magnetic field, which is responsible for life. It's the same thing with us.

There are techniques and methodologies that are formulas from wise people. They can totally turn you away from all kinds of dangers. The point is that God is perfect, omnipresent and omniscient. Whatever you want to call him. He can't create something that's incomplete. We are complete for the purposes of longitude and latitude, circumstances and confrontation. But why can't we live that way? Because we don't trust ourselves. Forget about trusting somebody else. If you don't trust yourself, how will you trust somebody else? If you don't love yourself, how can you love somebody else? If you don't talk to yourself, why would you talk to others?

Talk to yourself first. Let yourself know before you let anybody else know. I know I have to move the energy. This is class. This is what you want. This is what I have to deliver. Have you seen me stopping until I am sure it's a done deal? The job has to be done. It has to be. If I have to do it, I have to do it.

In your deliverance lies the ecstasy. In your deliverance lies your bounty. In your deliverance lies your bliss. In your deliverance lies your beauty. Everything else will fall short. Learn to deliver. Deliver yourself to your body, yourself to your mind. There are two aspects to deal with: let your soul talk to your mind and let your soul talk to your body. And let yourself know your soul. All matters will be adjusted. All things will be taken care of. It's as simple as that.

Challenges are inevitable. You can't avoid them. Come and go, up and down shall happen. You don't want to face it? Be yourself.

Keep your *sadhana*.[41] Keep yourself intact. As long as you keep yourself in one piece, you will have peace of mind. Just remember—all prosperity comes through peace. If you keep yourself in one piece, you will be fine. Don't love God out there somewhere. Love God within you. This outside God is a lie. It's a betrayal. It's a treachery. There is no such thing as anything beyond you.

What is in you, that's all that God is about.

> *In your deliverance lies your ecstasy.*
>
> *In your deliverance lies your bounty.*
>
> *In your deliverance lies your bliss.*
>
> *In your deliverance lies your beauty.*
>
> *Everything else will fall short.*
>
> *Learn to deliver.*

---

[41] *Sadhana*: daily spiritual practice. It can include prayer, yoga, meditation and chanting that you do to connect you to your spirit.

Chapter Twelve

Kindness Brings Prosperity

Reproductivity is part of the female—is that true? Anything more than one child is abundance. In the early times, people used to have six or eight children. There was no school then. They used to send each child to *Gurukul*, and the children would study, grow, become powerful and earn.

The female has a natural power of abundance, good luck, and prosperity, if she decides to concentrate on it. If a woman provokes the Divine, there is no reason that she will not be prosperous. Her discipline guarantees it. A woman with good manners concentrates on the very item of prosperity. And what is that? What is prosperity? She expands herself through goodwill, good manners, smiles, counseling and uplifting. Whenever a woman puts all these good things together, prosperity in abundance is assured.

But as a female, if she wastes her time betraying, yelling, screaming, calling names and being rude, poverty is assured. For a female health, wealth and happiness lie in her manners.

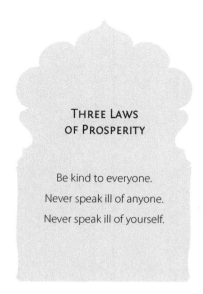

**THREE LAWS
OF PROSPERITY**

Be kind to everyone.

Never speak ill of anyone.

Never speak ill of yourself.

You can study in many colleges and do anything. Basically, it will come down to one thing: kindness, a woman making it her priority to be kind. Kindness is an essential part of every female. And in kindness, as you expand, prosperity will come with it. You will have more friends. You will have more opportunities. Good luck will knock at your door. Why? Because you are kind, compassionate and you have good manners. Everything that you call prosperity rests on it.

They say a woman can make a palace out of a straw house.

On this planet, the only mammal that can change life is the female. She has X amount of energy. If she doesn't waste that energy in many different directions, and if she concentrates in one way and means it, then there is nothing that can stop her from becoming prosperous. You must meet people. You must receive people. You must talk to people. You must share your wisdom with people. There are one hundred and eight elements in this universe. All of that is at the tip of your fingers, provided you decide to be compassionate, kind and caring.

Now what can stop you? The idea is to just stop. Just wait—don't react. Just don't react. There lies the whole universe if you just don't react. All the energy we waste being jealous, being neurotic, talking negatively, competing and comparing in a very negative way—these are not essential things in life. Let us see, in our goodness, how good we can be.

My grandmother used to make butter in the morning. She would read, by memory, the five *banis*[42] and then give us butter. If we recited them correctly with her, then she would give us Gud, candy. Otherwise no. There was a vibration, a relationship.

Your children are your children if you feed them your *prana*. Use your own hands and feed yourself if you cannot feed your children. Peel the banana and feed your husband so he may not be negative. If you cannot be affectionate with each other then the result will be negative.

These are serious things. How many of you have gone to have lunch with a friend and fed a friend just one bite or so?

What has happened to that thing called affection?

You women—you are the source of life. You are the source of life. You are the life.

Sometimes you are so crazy, you even split God into male and female. God is neither male nor female. If God is male then it must be in the post office.

There is no good and bad. I am not kidding. There is no guilt. There is no sin. There is no wrong. There is no right. It's our own insanity and our own meditative concentration.

So what is God? Male, female, crazy, wise, Jew, Muslim? God is a living energy. It lives in you.

The first principle of life is if you are a human, you should be loving. That's the rule of thumb. Love first, everything will come to you.

---

[42] *Banis*: Traditional daily prayers in *Sikh Dharma*.

WHAT IS?[43]

What is business? Negotiations.

What is the hub of life? Mutuality.

What is the fragrance of life? Never let down.

What is poverty? Going for things.

What is royalty? Letting it come to you.

What is man's greatest asset? Manners.

What is the worst thing that can happen to you?
Loose your cool.

What is everyman afraid of? Tomorrow.

What is prosperity? Delivery and deliverance.

Who will take care of me? Me, myself and I.

Excuses are self-abuses.

---

[43] © The Teachings of Yogi Bhajan, August, 21, 1996

CHAPTER THIRTEEN

SUCCESS IN BUSINESS

The basic subject today is "Interlog of the interest—human, monetary, and personal." The subject is extremely boring and everybody hates to deal with it. It's so hate-worthy that we put many names on it and size up its potential in many ways. But without this, no business can sustain itself—none.

The difference between a business and a government is that when a government goofs, they can pass a revised budget. The first budget they call an interim budget. The revised is called a supplementary budget. First the main budget is passed, and then they create a supplementary budget. When a government passes a supplementary budget it means it has goofed on the interlog. The interest interlog was not considered. Whoever made the budget is just a creep. Now, what is there to do? The government has to come through. There are two ways for a government to do this: 1) print money—which leads to inflation or 2) tighten the money—and then industries collapse. Instead, the government comes out with a supplementary budget.

It may surprise you that in all democracies, you will find a supplementary budget, but in domestic life, this is not possible. As a business, it is possible in the sense that you can ask a bank for more money and a longer credit line. But a bank will not be nice to you if you do not have a tremendous amount of collateral and a wonderful record. So it's a very thin line.

What is this all about? Where do we goof? What are the slips and the pits? How we can cover ourselves? That's the subject that I want to go into with you.

We are the center of the business. The center of the business is not the office. It's not administration. It's not management. It's not the billboard outside. It's not the secretary inside. It's not the reception room. It's not the person, his suit, his coat or his brooch. It is in the head.

The center of the business is that somewhere he is a C and there is a B and then we build a lot of paraphernalia around it. We proceed and start building something small. Then it becomes big—so big that it takes over. And it can go on and on and on and on.

One business takes over another business, which takes over another business. Every business has to have a strategy. Every strategy has to have a projection. It is like a romantic relationship, but it is extremely boring because in romance you have another person to play with. In business, you have to have another business to play with.

Once I said to somebody, "You are a multi-multi-millionaire. You have so many businesses that you can't even list them. Why do you want more businesses?"

He said, "Just for the more of it."

If you don't have that attitude, "I want more. I want more. I want more of the more," then you can't handle it. Life will become painful, and you will be absolutely small.

Remember, in the business world, that the little fish is always eaten by the big fish. They always say the little fish is a meal for the big fish. Don't take it wrong. Ultimately in this ocean of business, the only thing that survives is not the business. It is you. The business is your projection. The business is your reflection. The business is your identity and the business is an institution to which you can do two things. In an institution you can either live off the institution or you can live out of it.

You can be lazy. You can delay. You can think wrong. Your projections can fail. That is why in business they say, "Watch 'I.'"

What does it mean to "Watch 'I'?" Write the interlog. L-O-G. It is the daily log of your business. They call it *rokad*.

You must understand—the first business center of the world was India and they have a language called *Landey*. You don't have to lift a pen writing the entire business sequence. One kind of line means one million dollars. Another kind of line means minus a million dollars. A little twist in it means nothing. A little twist the other way means everything. It's a complete language. But in that language you do not lift your pen—you continue and the language is called *Landey*.

If you look at *Landey* the writing looks like snail lines. You can't understand what it is all this about. But it's a business record. It's a journal of the business. In the western world, we call it a daily journal. In the original language, it's called *rokad*.

Every day, you write and hold yourself accountable to the business, like a daily diary. What did I do today? What are my fears? What are my threats? What are my projections? What are my goals? What are my achievements? What do I want to achieve? What have I achieved?

You are afraid to do that because you are afraid to be exposed. But why are you afraid to be exposed, but not afraid to be dumped? You have a choice between the two.

In the daily journal, this is what you have to watch out for. Every day you must know your investments. Every day, in those investments, you must know your current expenses. Every day you must know your projected expenses. And every day you must know your Reserve Power to Meet Expenses. RPME. We always say, "rip me." Because once this reserve power doesn't meet the expenses, you have bad news.

In the business world you can give lip service; you can be appreciated; you can be talked to; you can romance; you are beautiful. But when it comes to RPME, it's a matter of weeks, days or months. Your boat is on the rocks and this figure must tell you where you stand.

In this fluctuation, you can increase your credit line and feel comfortable. You can get investors. You can get partners. Or you can go on a rampage—merge, submerge, ask, don't ask. If you read the *Wall Street Journal*, you will find this is an everyday affair. It was no different thousands of years ago, and it is not going to be any different thousand of years from now. This is the vital link of a working life and a business life.

Business has certain rules. You want to know them? Here is Ms. B. Ms. B has a lover and Ms. B has a villain.

The villain is a frustrated lover who wants it but can't get it. The villain is never a good person. So Ms. B has a lover and a villain, and they have names. Mr. Profit and Mr. Loss.

These are the two polarities that are romancing, advancing, sending flowers, throwing arrows, throwing stones, creating goodwill and creating bad will all the time. It's a constant process and it will never end as long as the business will live.

The problem with you is you do not want to play this romance. But Ms. B does. Her dating capacity is fixed. You can match it or you can't match it. If you can't match it you are out of business. If you can match it, you are in business. In and out is decided right there.

Now, profit has support. The first support is goodwill. The second is bank will. The third is consumer's will. And the fourth is opportunity—chain stores, big accounts and all that rigmarole. That is why we do PR.

Her losses on the villain side are bad management, bad temper, bad judgment and bad PR. But the bottom line is good products over bad products. If it is a good product, you will survive even if the villain is all-in and you are not making sense. But if it's a bad product, you don't have a chance.

They say in real estate there are three things: location, location, location. In business, it is product, product, product. If the consumer needs the product and you have the right mind for it, the right opportunity for it, then you can sell it—your business can go on. But you have to watch your daily journal. The business cannot survive if you do not watch this. In your daily calculation there are certain do's. Every day you should know what interest you are paying; what administrative cost you have added or deleted; what commissions and commitments you are making today to further the business; what are your projected expenses; whether you are spreading your self too thin or you are solid.

The tragedy of business is that we only start thinking about these things when we are confronted with problems. That's not the way to do it. Business has to be recorded daily; in your daily journal put all these points clearly before you.

Every day, you have to see income, projected income, the analysis report, matching goals, contacts, expansion and new territories. In business, if you do not entertain new territories, new thoughts and new blood, you may be successful but you will be out of the field. No business by itself can sustain itself. You are spiritual people, and I tell you even God couldn't live in His own boredom. He had to expand. You have to get out, get new ideas, new territories, new contacts. You have to have something, one thing or another. The end is endless.

In business, just remember one line: The end is endless.

ਅੰਤ ਬੇਅੰਤੁ ਹੈ

Ant beyant hai.

If you can maintain that psychological mentality and not mess around with small things, you have a perfect attitude for business. If you can't, just consult.

The most dangerous thing in business, of which everybody is a victim, is the internal audit. Every government has an internal audit. Every good business has an internal audit. Every company has an internal audit. Planning cannot be based on your point of view, your bank support or your possibilities. It has to be based on the internal audit report.

The strength of a business is shown in the internal audit report. It cannot be imaginative. It cannot be subjective. It cannot be projective. The internal audit will tell you two and two.

And if you think in business you don't need the goodwill of people, you don't need PR of the people; if you don't want to send presents and receive presents, you don't want to do all that—then you are out of business. Business is a continuous romance with the people you hate the most. Your human capacity is that you will romance the people you like the most. But in the business world you romance the people you hate the most. Send a present to somebody who is going to complain about you six months from now. That present can shut him up. It is called pre-confronting syndrome. Every client has it.

Watch your interests. Don't watch your interests by a profit table. Don't watch your interests in how you are expanding. It is called cataloging the interest logs, wherever your interests are. How are you serving? Serving clients, public relations, the future, friends, the bank, your wife, your children, your car.

A bad car can have a flat on your way somewhere and you can miss an appointment. Your wife can create a stir at lunch or at breakfast and then you will not have a good day even though you have a business meeting. Your child can goof up in school and create an emergency. Create a trauma. Create a drama. You can deliver the wrong present to the right person and right present to the wrong person. This is called human error. To avoid human error, you need an executive secretary—a male or a female—the choice of gender is yours.

In the business world, the worst thing is that the one person you do not want to listen to is the executive secretary. When the executive secretary speaks, a businessman thinks his mother is talking.

There are two most tragic things in a business: individuality and authority. We all say in business, "I want to do the business." Actually, the business wants to do you. You can never do a business if you want to do a business. If you let the business do you, you are in business. If you let the business do you, you will become a specialist. You will become an expert. You will become somebody. When you want to do business, it will be only you and nothing more.

One Colombian emerald was found and sold for nine thousand dollars. It was cut and set into a necklace. The necklace sold for eleven million dollars. There were only three people in that business. One had the eye to know it, the other had the eye to cut it, and the third one had the eye to jewel it. The customers were there.

Have you heard the story about a man who bought two stones. They happened to be sapphires. He rounded them up, and sold them for millions of dollars. This man thought he was the

> ### FIVE POINTS TO REMEMBER IN THE BUSINESS WORLD
>
> 1. When work speaks, people go silent in reverence.
> 2. Every head bows to legacy not lineage.
> 3. You have no right if you are not all right.
> 4. Business is best by itself. Serve it—it will score for you. Shirk it—it will throw you out.
> 5. There should not be any conflict between your job and you. Be conscious of it.

best. Somebody else took those sapphires and rounded it up better and brought the gem quality out of them. He sold them for six hundred percent more. In that one deal, a town was built.

You can sell a trainload of mung beans and rice or you can sell one diamond. The question is the commission.

Business is nothing but a polite, democratic hysteria. It's an avalanche. It puts you out. Either you have to go under or you have to run. If you can run away with it, you make it. But there are certain practical aspects of business you must understand. Every business has an identity and it has to be served by a certain caliber. Not by your friendships. Not by your likes. Not by your dislikes.

Now watch yourself. Go inside and find out how many of you are willing to make friends in business when you know that those people are your sworn enemies. But business is business. You have to watch the interests of business over your own interests. Your personal interests, personal likes, personal habits, personal projection, personal dreams, personal relationships—all that is. Just remember, the business also has interests. The choice is: do you want to let the business win or do you want to win? If you want to win, the business will destroy you and itself. If you let the business win, you may get destroyed along the way, but the business will live. That's the only choice. That's why great businessmen die of a heart attack at a young age.

The daily diary, daily journal, writing the daily log of the interests of the business is essential. It is a very boring practice. It's cumbersome. And the daily log of your business practices, called *rokad,* must match up with the internal audit. If it doesn't, then within one week, a deadline has to be set to take out the bugs. Otherwise, you are dead. That is how sophisticated business problems are.

If you want to just build your individual ego and call it a business; if you want to just show off your individuality and call it a business; and if you just want to boast about something that you fell into through luck and call it a business; then you are out of business. You are "showbiz." You can go on for a while, but you won't last. Business is an everlasting process of life. It can go on with you. It can go on without you. Your importance in the business world is only whether you are with it or not.

I knew a businessman who used to do a commodity business. His range was sixty to seventy million dollars a day. If one day he lost seventy million dollars, the next day he would make sixty million dollars. If one day he made a hundred and seventy million dollars, he would feel lucky. Then, he could lag behind for three days. Every day it was back and forth.

He started goofing up because he had a desire to retire, but he couldn't. He was a single man who never trained anybody, who never shared with anybody. All he had was himself and his secretary. When his business started crumbling, he took about two hundred and some friends with him. He started calling the bank, and the bank had a such a good record with him for thirty or forty years, they were willing to extend him anything. When he phoned his friends and asked, they gave to him. And everything went down with it. It was the biggest earthquake that nobody saw coming—nobody knew. And those painful hearts are still bleeding. That can happen to anybody.

Therefore, please remember the interest of the business is based on one line. You can fail. The business can fail, but the system cannot fail. Make a system and just understand that this is a triangle. There are three points: there is you; there is the business profit and identity; and there is your projection—the future, your ego, call it anything. But in the center, there is the eye. It must keep on seeing all aspects.

Just remember to watch the interests of the business. Don't read into the business. Read the words on the wall that the business is telling you. And don't ever feel afraid to investigate what's going on. Normally, when a business starts telling us it's not good, we patch it up or cover it up. We don't want it to be known because our ego is involved. Remember, a business has its own ego. It has nothing to do with you. It's just providing you an opportunity.

HOW LONG DOES IT TAKE FOR A BUSINESS TO MAKE A PROFIT?

The first year, you open the shop. The second year, you pay for the shop from the capital. You work your investment into it. And the third year, it should start making a profit.

The first year people get to know you. You get to do it. The shelves are made, the store is bought, thing happen, etc. That's the first year. You don't know anything.

The second year is chati. Chati means your principal is going out. And the third year, it starts making the interest back. That's a good business.

If you cater to ten percent of the population or twenty percent of the population, you have to be extremely fast and telescopically and microscopically correct. Otherwise, have a business for the general population. In business, it's a choice between eighty percent of the population or twenty percent of the population. Special businesses—small businesses and all that—serve the eighty percent. If you focus on twenty percent, you can serve five percent, ten percent or total twenty percent of the population. You don't have a big choice. The range of customers is very limited in the upper hemispheres.

Many businesses are run by men who leave them to the woman they think they love the most. But a lot of men are corrupt, shady and inferior. They do not enjoy the business. So their mastery is in ruling the world and keeping the slave, called a woman. Ultimately it is an M, opposite of that is a W. In that juggling, the whole world moves.

You will find in the real business world that there are men who are successful and then leave the businesses to their wives. They still live. Who runs the businesses? The accountants, the administrators and everything do. The men who started the businesses, worked for it and did everything, are gone. For a male, it is very difficult to cater to the ego of the business—to share it and put the structure right, to watch the interest and carry it thoroughly.

Normally the beasts of burden, those who sweat and labor are males, not females. If you put a woman into a business, she is so sharp and cutthroat that you don't have a chance against her. A woman in business will guard it like a mother guards her child. Her whole sensitivity will come into play. That's why, in business, if you have a good executive secretary you are very protected and safe.

You need a business attitude. Look at Hindus. I like that religion very much. They go to the shop. They will not sit on the chair, they will put the battis (Hindu chants) on, and they will worship the business. They will worship Shiva, the God of death, Vishnu the God of providing, and Brahma, the God of opportunities and originality. They will put Ganesha there for good luck. They will not put any family pictures or anything. And they will worship it as an altar.

At night, when they close their daily account, they always write a personal note—always. The personal note concludes what they have done with the business that day. If you meet a successful Indian businessman and tell him to come, he will say, " Five minutes." You know what that means? He wants to pray for five minutes to himself. It is their common way of behavior. Five minutes. You always wonder what's wrong with these guys? Five minutes—what does he want with five minutes? Those five minutes are his—between him and his business intelligence.

Have a System that Works

As far as business is concerned, if your employee has stolen, you should put all your trust in him because your system has failed. Employees always steal. There's no reason why not. Where did they tell you employees won't steal? Haves and have-nots always fight. You have. He doesn't have. He must steal.

Everybody steals everybody's husband. Everybody steals everybody's child. Everybody steals everybody's business. Everybody steals from everybody. The world is full of thieves.

ਅਸੰਖ ਚੋਰ ਹਰਾਮਖੋਰ ॥
ਅਸੰਖ ਅਮਰ ਕਰਿ ਜਾਹਿ ਜੋਰ ॥

Asankh chor haraam khor.
Asankh amar kar jaahi jor.

Countless the thieves who make their living by exploiting others.
Countless who use power in the service of their own egos.

— Guru Nanak, *Japji Sahib*, Pauree18

Guru Nanak said it. Don't you read *Japji* in the morning? Uncountable thieves. *Asankh chor, haraamkhor*. There are uncountable thieves.

Everybody in business steals. Business is a glorified and classified thievery. What do you do? You buy cheap and you sell high, right? And you get somebody's money. You call it profit. What is it? If the other guy could go to the store where you got it, he would go and get it there.

If you tell somebody that the factory price is twenty dollars, and the consumer price is a hundred and twenty dollars, see how many times he buys it. No. Instead you tell him that it's a hundred and fifty dollars, but I am giving it to you for a hundred and twenty dollars. You see the signs, "Sale! Sale! Sale!" What is this sale? Jack up the price three times and reduce it to one third? Is that not thievery?

What's goodwill? Goodwill is just polishing somebody so he keeps his eyes closed.

Once in our business I had a subordinate. He was just a pain-in-the-neck idiot who never dealt with anything right. Never. Finally they told him, if you can just have one room opposite the garden and just watch the garden, we'll pay your salary. Nobody wanted him. Nobody wanted to talk to him. But nobody could dismiss him except me, and I wouldn't touch it.

So the matter went on and on and on, and almost everybody wrote him off. When everybody wrote him off, he would come and ask, "Hello, sir. Hello. Do you have any job for me?" And I would say, "No, I am satisfied. You can go." And he would go wherever he wanted to go.

Four years later, I called him into my office. He sat down. I said, "Well you have not wasted four years. You have nurtured yourself. You have recuperated yourself, and you have enjoyed yourself." I didn't say, "You just got paid for nothing, you son of this and this." No, I put a positive note on it myself and I said, "You did everything wonderfully. But now we have a very special job and there is nobody else who can do it." And I handed over to him a sealed paper with a red ribbon.

He said, "What do I have to do?"

I said, "If you do it, you will come back and I will thank you. If you get lost along the way, adios. But only you can do this job."

Patience paid. After four years, his entire intelligence and concentration came in handy. He just wanted to prove that he could do it. And I knew nobody else would even have the guts to touch this request. He came through.

So you can never know who will come through in business. Keep your options open. Keep your eyes open. Keep your ears open and keep your system strong.

Everybody said, "Why did you give him a garden room?"

I said, "So we can look at what he's doing. Everybody passes through the gardens. Everybody looks at the window and the door. There are glass windows."

That's why in banks, they don't have rooms but those dividers. In between the dividers, they provide windows. The idea is nobody should goof up. This is a system. Let everything fail, but not the system. You will never regret it.

Employees do steal. But it means your system is not right. Your inventory is not right. Your audit is not right. Things are not right.

There is a simple game. Everybody wants your money, honey. There are three things everybody wants to share: your power of money, your domain and your status. That's what business is about.

Politics is what? Status. They spend three million dollars for a job that pays twenty thousand dollars. It's not worth the interest. They go door to door begging, asking friends to pay for it. What is a political donation? Asking for money with a promise to serve later. You think it is not stealing? Have you seen any man in an election campaign who doesn't go door to door and shake hands even with those who have not washed their hands? But when they get elected—ask them to shake hands.

You are ill without skill. Skill is when you put the sky to the ill, then it becomes skill. It's called being an expert, a specialist. If your business won't fail, you may fail, but you still keep going. That's why we humans want businesses—to keep us busy. Business and opportunity will never wait for you. That's a common mistake we all commit. We think business will wait for us. No way. Business and opportunity never wait for anybody. You've got to cash it.

RISK AND SUCCESS

Without risk, there is no business. And if the risk is more than you, there is no business. So when you have a potential, play it out. That's where partnership, corporation and sharing all came in. When people found out that it's not possible to have partners, it's difficult to have partners, they started making corporations. They said, we cannot sit together and have a partnership, but let us create a corporation. Let the interest live. What is a corporation? Business interest.

A good business should give you between ten to twenty percent net profit. That's a very lucrative, good business. If it steadily gives you five to seven percent, it's not bad. When it starts being less than that, your planning is wrong. If after five years, the business matches up to zero, there is something seriously wrong. If in two years you do not expand the business, there is something wrong with your head. If in one year you do not plan to expand, there is something wrong with your heart. It's an organism. It keeps going. There's no end to it. The organic world stops for nothing.

The business world has its own theory. "I am busy. See me later." No. You have to see that person right there and then. And for that, you have to take a flower with a fragrance that suits the opportunity. That's why in the business world they say never present yourself without a present. Because you won't attract anything. Your present will. Some special present combined with your presence will create the dialogue.

There is a common saying: weak men and a good business make a bad combination. It's none of my business but King Edward the Eighth left the throne and an entire generation just for some idea called, "the biggest love in the world." So who knows who wants to do what?

Basically, business is nothing but busy-ness to expand and secure. Along with that, there is always an interest to scare yourself and to commit your own death. They go hand in hand—especially in the western world. You come from a very cutthroat society because you have not been conceived in love; you have not been raised in love; and you have never been dealt with with love. Your love is to go and get. The question is, what do you think you go and get?

In the western world, our government pays million and millions of dollars in martial aid, in this aid, in that aid. But do we have a friend in the UN? We have to use our veto every time. Have you seen the Russians? They are oriental. They never pay anybody anything. They get the cash first, even to give arms. They never use their veto and they never give martial aid to anybody. Their only mistakes—they walked into Afghanistan and they walked into Cuba. It cost Russia seventeen million dollars a day to keep us ninety miles away and the island alive.

Remember one thing: business is not a puppetry of emotions. It's not a drama of feelings. And it's not a drama of ego. Business is a pure sense of purity. It's very meditative living if you really want to know. The reality is you have to be one step ahead.

Let us put it in small example. A husband and a wife have a store. They live on the top story. They come downstairs for the shop. They open it on time, they smile at everybody, they keep the goodwill in the neighborhood and they have the goods. Do you understand? Take this small business. See how calm, serene, good and moral it is.

There is a very popular saying: "With business, we can live. Without business, we do not know why we are living." If you know why you are living, then have a business. I have seen a syllabus from a graduate business course and I was surprised by what they teach. I think what they teach is not business, but mostly mannerisms—how you can go and get it. And if there are thirty or forty opportunities and you get one, then you are done. That's not business either. That's why in America more businesses fail per hundred than continue. The rate of collapse is tremendous here. People freak out. They get isolated and segregated. There's no expansion, no new ideas. People are scared to death—they can't share, can't relax, can't plan, can't go bigger, can't become more energized and they can't become more radiant. They are afraid to have personal contact.

Do you want to write down the saying of the day?

"Without a smile, business is a mile away."

Here is one of the worst tragedies that ever happened. Somebody went to the bank, and presented his business proposal. They discussed the whole thing and the bank said, "Yes. How much do you want?"

The man said, "A five- to six-million-dollar credit line and three million dollars now in advance. It's an eleven-million-dollar project. We'll start with eight million dollars." The bank said yes. All the papers were signed. Everything was fine, wonderful.

Three months later, the bank folded up and the credit line went with it.

You have to be ready for an eventual unexpected remote possibility. That's why in business, the system has to be right.

The guy called me up. He said, "The bank is gone. I am in the middle of the project. Is there any spiritual way to look at it?"

I said, "Yes. How many customers do you have? How many sale orders have you got? How many this and that?"

I said, "Write a letter to everybody and tell them the bank has folded. I am going to fold also unless you can send me your credit line, then I can make it and I will give you a twenty percent discount in the end."

He is still in business. It worked very well. His promises were not great. His labor was very sweaty. He was expecting to make forty percent. He ended up making ten percent. But you know, he survived. If you have done your homework, then you have done well. You are not wrong. Nobody loves anybody. They go for the profit.

On this planet, in the business world, nothing sells but specialty. You have to be special. Once I asked somebody "What's your specialty?"

He said, "I am a potato chopper."

"What is that?"

"Give me a potato and I will show you."

I gave him a wooden board, a potato and a knife. You can't believe what he did with that potato. He made flowers out of it. He made a bullock cart. He made a wagon. With all those toothpicks and potatos and a knife, the guy created a line of art. Back in those days in Canada, asking ten dollars an hour was a lot of money. He had nine offers. He could cut a potato to the point of art. When you sell a potato, you make five cents. If you cut a potato, you will make ten bucks.

The difference is between surviving and being an artist. The process of life is constantly graduating from one level to the next.

You must learn to watch the interest. And the only way you can watch the interest of your business is if you log your interest. Interlogging the interest is the capital word for all the details in your business that you want to know.

HIRING AND FIRING

When you hire somebody, you invest a lot. You know the habits of that person. You know the weaknesses. You know a lot of stuff, and it's a very good cozy situation.

In time, firing is possible. But firing someone in a quick manner is losing the last opportunity. The best way to fire somebody is to squeeze him or her to the point that he says adios himself or herself. Because work, itself, has a demand. And when the demand of the work does not tell the employee to quit, it means your system is not right. Your system will squeeze people out and the fittest will survive. Why should you fire anyone? The wind will take them away.

I am always willing to take a thirty percent loss on the gross of an individual because I know they are not going to come through. They are not going to make it. From day one, I always include that in my planning. Do you understand what I mean? I don't expect a person to arrive at nine o'clock and perform until five o'clock with a missionary's zeal. And if someone does perform with a missionary's zeal, do you think he's not going to make thirty blunders? I don't believe that. So I am ready to be cut both ways. It's as simple as that. If I know the person is honest, that he wants to work, that he wants to produce, I also know that while he's doing it, he is going to get a lot of tickets—traffic tickets. Or I know that the person is so slow, I have to hire someone to push him to keep on going. But that's a net thirty percent.

There is no hiring and firing, to be honest. Put the company first. Put the identity first. Put the business interest first. We are not successful because we don't do that. We deal with business very emotionally. Not simply.

So my personal feeling is never hire anybody, never fire anybody, let everybody come in and work it out. If you have a good workout, and the person can sweat—fine. If he gets tired and doesn't show up the next morning—what good luck. I know the answer you want but I have to give the answer that I believe in.

So the normal approach is that when a person is not cost-effective, disciplined or PR-effective, fire him right away before lunch happens.

But I don't know what firing means, actually. Because if you fire a rifle and you do not know how to zero the rifle, you will miss the buck. Firing is a very heavy process. Hiring and firing is personnel management. It's the most difficult aspect of the entire business world. People have their personal personality, their conflicting personal projections and their interrelationships. Their demands are more. Their needs are more. They are different, and it does conflict with business all the time. The personal personality and the business personality always conflict—including with the owner.

So if you think firing is the way, have a firing department. Court-martial everybody. I don't know why one has to fire or hire anybody. I think it's all smooth. It takes years to become special.

RAISING CAPITAL AND BECOMING PROSPEROUS

Capital raising. Here are a few basic fundamentals. First is the spread. This is most important. If you spread it properly and paint the picture well, and if you give it to anyone with capital money, they will go for it. It's called the profile—the business profile of the business subject. That's the first, initial thing that you must prepare very well and at length.

You must know what you have. How you have it. What it can do for you. What it can do for others. What are the checks and balances? What is the security? What is the collateral? What is possible? What Wall Street has said. What the business journals say. The whole thing. If you make the packet properly, your scheme will work. Forget about collateral.

When you must go to somebody and ask for money, if you do not have the spread, then he must either be your father-in-law or your father. Otherwise without the spread, your chance to raise the capital is dead.

Business is done for nothing but security. Give the spread and the security, you will get the capital. The bank will give it to you. Because what does a bank want? A bank wants to invest the money. But they want to invest it on very solid grounds.

In a business, if you are not in touch with the impulse of the money market, you are out. You've got to know what is going on in the money market, what the trends are, and what is happening.

You have to work with the transmission of the trend, and the trend must be predicted. It's called marketing. Marketing is nothing but the predictable possibilities of the future, the present and the past. It's the total history. It gives you the geography of the business.

I knew 3HO didn't have money. I knew *Dasvand* was down. I knew the whole problem and I saw the figures. So I asked Sada Sat Singh, "Can I teach?"

He said, "Yes. We'll give you two days."

I got the two days. And I knew if I were to teach, I would fill the class. I fill the class because I know my commodity is good. I teach good. I am not good, do you understand? I am a businessman. I am not good and I don't care if I am good or bad. But I know what I teach is priceless. I sell wherever I am.

Don't promise people what you can't deliver. You can take one chance, but the second time, nobody will trust you. My idea is very simple. In business, blow up everything but don't blow up the trust of somebody. It hurts deeper, talk spreads faster and bad will will overcome you like an avalanche. Don't ever do it. There are a lot of people in the world who want to share with you, if they understand you are a solid person. You look solid, that's fine. You have solid practices, it's fine. If the business is solid and your habits are solid, they will go for it.

Quackery is not business and emotional nonsense doesn't make any sense. Once, somebody wanted to go and meet the president of the bank. He had a good scheme, a wonderful idea, and he had an account with that bank for the last twenty years. He was the main client. So he said, "Okay, I will go and meet a friend."

He went to meet the president of the bank. They gave him a royal entrance. He went into the room and saw the president of the bank crying and he couldn't believe it. He said, "George, what happened?"

The bank president replied, "I O.D.'d last night."

He said, "I am sorry. I am very grateful to you. I came. Thank you very much for your time. Would you like to talk to me?"

The bank president said, "No, I will come later."

The bank lost the account, the business and a friend—three in one stroke. The board of directors came to know about it and they fired the president.

The business world is a world unto itself. If you play in it, play with a smile or you don't belong to it. The world is very cutthroat.

Once somebody in his business hired somebody and he called to tell me about it. "Oh, la la."

I said, "Watch out with this guy."

"How come? His profile is this, his personality is this."

"Look, with this kind of profile and personality, the guy has come to you on this salary? It's impossible to believe. Either there is something he is not telling you, or something you are not aware of. Look deeply into it."

One year went by, the second year went by and there was no problem. We met, and he said, "Well, two years have gone by, I don't see the problem."

I said, "Sometimes these people take a long time to put you into a bondage of trust and then they kill you."

"Why would he do that?"

"It's a habit." I told him the story of the frog and scorpion. When the frog was in the center of the river, the scorpion bit him. The frog was dying and said, "Why did you do it?"

The scorpion said, "Because it's my habit."

The frog said, "But you are dying with me."

The scorpion said, "Well, that's my luck. I did what I have a habit to do."

So I told him, "There must be some habit. Check it out. Two years have gone by. That's enough."

"Yes sir."

He went back. He looked into the situation very thoroughly and he found it.

My feeling is the business must survive. The object is tomorrow, and tomorrow is there for us.

Sometimes you create a business where there's too much imagination, when very little practical homework has been done. And sometime you like it and love it so much, you don't want to let it move. Both are common tragedies. They are called unfair human practices.

I asked one guy, "Why didn't you call me before?"

He said, "I was afraid."

"Afraid of what? I'm not going eat you up. I am not going to take away your business. I don't care. If you make a million dollars, that's good for me."

What is my beauty? Look, if you make a million dollars and I come to your town, you will hire a limousine for me. You will take care of me and I will have fun. If I go to your town and you are poor, then you will try to find where my wallet is and you will like to steal it.

This is one thing I know. I came to the United States with thirty-five dollars in my pocket. Nobody has done me any favors. I have earned every buck of mine. I have paid every tax of mine. I built an empire and I am leaving it to you. Are you so blind and stupid that you can't see it? And now you are interested in clashing with me when I tell you to take over? You say, "Hey, what? Take over? There must be some trick." What trick am I playing? I am sixty years old and I've got to go. I am hanging in there because you don't want to take over.

Each one of you by your own right must have prosperity. Otherwise, Guru Nanak has gone wrong. He said, rise in the ambrosial hour—which you don't, but if you do … He said earn through the sweat of your brow—which you try to, but sometimes you don't. And then he said share. Now how can you share, if you have nothing? You want to share nothingness? It won't work. Giving is the grit of *Sikh Dharma*. It's the spirit of *Sikh Dharma*. Without it, *Sikh Dharma* dies. So we will keep giving. We cannot give if we cannot make it. And the fun of giving is to make it in abundance.

Chapter Fourteen

The Law of the Journey of the Soul

The soul has a journey, and it is pre-destined. It selects its longitude and latitude to be born. It selects its geography; its space; its protective, nurturing essence of the parents, mother and father; and its environments. All the aspects, all the events that happen in the first seven years are set. It is just like when you have a book. Let us say somebody has a sixty-page book that's called "Life." Every page has to be turned, and every page has to be read. Every page has to be gone through and has to be understood.

In between, there can be cross-references. In between, there will be things you highlight—the things you like. There will be things that bring tears to your life, and there will be things that are dreadful. Things that are right and things you think are wrong. So let us say life proceeds like a book. Every tomorrow will become today. There shall not be, nor should there be, a tomorrow in fear. But there should be a tomorrow in existence. Elementary tomorrow is already in existence. You have to walk on it.

I'm giving these examples so you can understand how life and the soul proceed in combination with the elements and the environments. Then no one will make a mistake.

Like a freeway, there are lanes, and you set out. There are set driving rules. There are set exits. There is a set number of miles you have to travel. If your car goes by the set rules and procedures, then it will travel the distance to the destination. But on the other hand, you can cause an accident. You can bump into another car. You can slip off the freeway. You can fall apart.

These accidents and coincidences also happen in life. Therefore, fundamentally what we require is a very clear consciousness. You require a windshield wiper in case of rain. You want to see the windshield is clear. You want to see clearly; you want to see what is coming in front of you. You have mirrors on the side. You want to see what is catching up with you and what you have left behind. You also have a mirror in front of you, and you want to look in the back to see what is going on. All of these aspects of the car in totality, that is *Ek Ong Kaar*. That is life. That is what you are. That is what *Naam* is.

Naam is the identity of your life in which you have traveled as the soul, looking left, right, front, sides and back. And then you have gauges before you—the speed, revolutions per minute, gasoline, temperature, water, etc. What I'm explaining is, we have things. If you fly an airplane, you will find a way to measure the longitude, latitude and height. You will find a huge number of buttons and meters to press and to watch. And then you will keep on going.

Everything that you control in the cockpit makes you the pilot of life. Exactly in your personal life, you are nothing more than a pilot, sitting in the cockpit, running the vehicle of the body through time on the vehicle of space. Going the distance from point A to point Z, where you have to continue to your destiny. This is how the soul travels. In between there can be an accident. There can be weather problems. There can be hazards in the way—the unexpected, the uncalled for, the unknown.

That's why consciousness is necessary. Some do not develop consciousness, but rather think, "Well, as the years will grow, we'll grow." That's why we need values. A pilot has to be tested. He has to go to a school. He has to be examined. He has to test pilot himself. That's why he's licensed, why he's certified.

Nobody ever was there to get you to where you are. You may have it, or you may not have it. You may go through it, or you may not go through it. You may travel through it or you may not travel through it. Nobody can decide for you. Suicide and completion of the journey are two sides of the coin.

Now, opportunities in life will give you the access, the exits. It will give you the essence of life. You can go wrong. You can go right. In our elements, age plays a part. Sometimes you are driving on the freeway, nice and clear, singing and dancing, and you are not fully aware of what you are doing. All of a sudden, the car stops, makes some noise, and nothing moves. What do you see? The parts fall apart. What will you do? Call Triple A, tow it to a mechanic, see what is happening, get it repaired, and it runs again.

But these incidents, coincidences, medical emergencies, good luck, bad luck—are all our expressions. Richness and poverty are all our expression. All of this is there. Nobody can wipe it out. But those who have consciousness and intelligence can enjoy it while going through it. Those who have not developed that consciousness and that clarity are subject to time and space. They do not enjoy life.

That's why our life starts in the ambrosial hours, early before the sun rises, and we prepare ourselves for each day. [44] We balance each day.

Similarly in life, there's one unison body. Wherever we are—we are one. We have not forgotten that in us there are three values: we are angels, we are humans and we are animals. Our barbaric animal nature is to live *at* each other. Our human nature is to live *with* each other. And our angelic nature is to live *for* each other. That should decide all our behavioral aspects. If we start looking at this Trinity, that is what our behavior is. If we teach our children these three fundamental natures and tell them the set rules for the angels, for the humans and for the barbarians, then we prepare them for life. And as we prepare them, we also get prepared. And as there is a child in us that also gets prepared, that child has to be fed, nurtured and educated every day, at every moment.

Whenever you decide to deal with somebody, ask yourself, "Am I an angel? Am I going to do it angelically? Am I doing it humanly? Am I going to be a brute—barbaric and neurotic?" This is very funny. For many, many years I have gone through time and space watching this. Actually, this is one movie I watch constantly. I see people—how they relate, how insecure they are. Watch them and see how insecure they are. See how nothing they are. When you show your commotions, see how nothing you are. When you show your commotions, you have absolutely no wisdom, no logic, no rational self and no faith left in you. You are just a confused self—a nothing.

Watch people. Watch people grabbing things. Watch people sticking to things. Watch their behavior and then you can understand. It is just like a leopard taking an animal and running it to the height of the tree to hide it. He killed it. He ate it. He wants it for tomorrow. That's animal nature. Look at the human. He will have one piece of bread. If somebody comes, he'll share it. Look at the angelic nature. He will look for somebody who's hungry and shall feed him or her. The human is the same. There are three natures always active, effective and working. This is the Age of Aquarius. This is the Age of Knowledge. "I know. I am."

Now, what is to be done? Am I going to adopt the behavior of an angel? Am I going to adopt the behavior of a human? Am I going to stay in my basic animal nature? Well, this is what I want to tell you. Tomorrow, after the completion of your journey, if your balance sheet says you have lived like an animal, you will go back into the animal nature. You will have the body of an animal, and you will be totally condemned to living an animal life.

If your behavior is as an unconscious animal, then you shall go to the sea world. You will never escape it. You will be living at each other. Look at the sea. Fish eats fish. They live at each other in a balance. They have absolutely nothing else to relate to. Look at the animals. They look, they eat. They eat, and they live. That's animal nature.

---

[44] In the practice of Kundalini Yoga and *Sikh Dharma*, the optimal time to do *sadhana*, the daily spiritual practice, is in the hours before sunrise. Normally considered to be 4-7 a.m.

If the balance sheet for this journey of life as a human shows insecurity, jealousy, greed and the unconclusive self; and if there is absolutely no positive, graceful, angelic nature; if there is no giving, then:

ਦੇਦਾ ਦੇ ਲੈਦੇ ਥਕਿ ਪਾਹਿ ॥
ਜੁਗਾ ਜੁਗੰਤਰਿ ਖਾਹੀ ਖਾਹਿ ॥
ਹੁਕਮੀ ਹੁਕਮੁ ਚਲਾਏ ਰਾਹੁ ॥
ਨਾਨਕ ਵਿਗਸੈ ਵੇਪਰਵਾਹੁ ॥੩॥

Daydaa day laiday thak paahi.
Jugaa jugantar khaahee khaahi.
Hukmee hukam chalaa-ay raahu.
Nanak vigsai vayparvaahu. ||3||

You, Great Giver, keep giving to us and we grow tired of just taking.
Age after age You continually feed and nourish us.
In Your Will, Oh Divine Spirit, You guide us along the path
You choose for us.
Nanak, blissful, hasn't a care.

— Guru Nanak, *Japji Sahib*, Pauree 3

Then you have no relationship to the fact that giving is the way of life. God gives, gives, gives, and gives; and we take, take, and get tired. Then you will never reincarnate as another human.

But if giving, sharing and loving; tolerating, kindness, compassion and caring is the nature, then at the end of this journey, the next life will only be human. Redemption is not there. Don't misunderstand, and don't tell me that I am *Dharam Raj*, the God of Judgment speaking. I know the science and I have seen it. I know how it happens. I'm just telling you how the journey of the soul is condemned by you and you alone. You put your soul into the depth of being in the sea or the animal world or the bird world. You do it. It is not that a human is born to go and reverse itself. It is when a human is born and acts that way. That is where the cycle of life goes negative and downward in its trend. And that is what I am trying to explain.

The second part is this. When you deal with kindness—comparative kindness, caring, and compassion—and you are nice and you go all the way to tolerate, be peaceful, educate others, be knowledgeable and clear minded, that next life gives you an improvement as a human.

But if you choose that you should be totally balanced, and you will only adopt the policy of God, which is to give, give, give because God gives; and God gives, gives, gives, gives and never gets tired. And you will never get tired of giving. Time after time after time after time He gives and gives and gives and gives. Time ends but God never ends His giving.

ਜੁਗਾ ਜੁਗੰਤਰਿ ਖਾਹੀ ਖਾਹਿ ॥
ਹੁਕਮੀ ਹੁਕਮੁ ਚਲਾਏ ਰਾਹੁ ॥

Jugaa jugantar khaahee khaahi.
Hukmee hukam chalaa-ay raahu.

Age after age You continually feed and nourish us.
In Your Will, Oh Divine Spirit, You guide us along the path You choose for us.

— Guru Nanak, *Japji Sahib*, Pauree 3

That carefree Lord moves like the wind, like a breeze in the morning, touching and kissing everybody, hugging, laughing and smiling through the angelic nature. If you become that kind of giver, you will become God. This is what Guru Nanak said in *Japji*. And that is what is understood.

Don't have a deep misunderstanding and commotional environments in which you think there is something else. That somebody outside is going to come and just touch your forehead and redeem you.

On this planet you can destroy yourself by excuses, by lies, by non-realistic existence, by fears, by comparative study and by an absolutely compassionate neurosis in which your "I," the ego, only extends to beyond any concept.

In that bitter fight, you are absolutely in a battle to the death in which you destroy your achievement as a human, which you have achieved now.

With the Guru's personal blessing,

ਗੁਰ ਸੇਵਾ ਤੇ ਭਗਤਿ ਕਮਾਈ ॥
ਤਬ ਇਹ ਮਾਨਸ ਦੇਹੀ ਪਾਈ ॥
ਇਸ ਦੇਹੀ ਕਉ ਸਿਮਰਹਿ ਦੇਵ ॥
ਸੋ ਦੇਹੀ ਭਜੁ ਹਰਿ ਕੀ ਸੇਵ ॥੧॥

Gur sayvaa tay bhagat kamaa-ee.
Tab ih maanas dayhee paa-ee.
Is dayhee ka-o simrahi dayv.
So dayhee bhaj har kee sayv. ||1||

You meditated and you did "*bhagatee,*" devotion.
Then you got this body. This body you got with all these concepts.
This body is 'worshipped by the angels.
With this body, do God's service.

Bhagat Kabir ji, *Siri Guru Granth Sahib,*
page 1159, line 7, as translated by Yogi Bhajan

"Har kee sev." God's service. Serve everybody who comes your way; touch everybody who comes your way; inspire everybody who comes your way; heal everybody who comes your way. Be nice, kind and compassionate to everybody who comes your way.

Just remember, every soul is a God and every soul is a test for you. Every soul is testing how you're behaving; how you're reacting; how you're projecting; how your aggression and progression is. Are you lying? Are you scared? What's your relationship?

I watch within myself every day. People forget who am I because they forget who they are personally. First you forget who you are, then you always forget who somebody else is. And with this forgetful nature, you forget everything. In this losing, forgetful nature, you lose everything, and the daily loss is accounted for. It's called the "balance sheet." In the end, there will be a panorama show where you will see everything you have done to protect yourself; where you have lied about yourself; all you have done to just ignore others, and hurt others.

So many people hurt me, left and right. So many people exert at each other left and right. So many people tell you left and right, "I'm your *wife*!" Then what? "I'm your *child*!" Then what? Are you a human? No. You are a wife, you are a son, you are a daughter, you are a person, you are a friend, you are an enemy. You are all these brands. When are you going to be human? If you are not ever going to be human, are you ever going to be a lover?

The frequency of the existence of the psyche has come into existence in love. It has not come into existence in protection and hatred. It has not come into existence to collect and grab everything around it. It is given environments by the will of God. Its co-existence is the glory of God. Its radiation and radiance are both by the spirit of God. Therefore, personally undermining someone creates indignity and insubordination to that higher principle—and it is a curse.

When are you going to be angelic? Are you a wife-angel, are you a wife-animal or are you a wife-human? Are you a son-angel, are you a son-human or are you a son-what? Daughter-what? Friend-what? These three identical natures are called "brands" in which we have to understand, study, divide and educate ourselves by our consciousness. It is called "applied conscious living."

ਮਨ ਤੂੰ ਜੋਤਿ ਸਰੂਪੁ ਹੈ ਅਪਨਾ ਮੂਲੁ ਪਛਾਣੁ ॥੫॥

Man toon jot saroop hai apnaa mool pachhaan. ||5||

Oh my mind, you are the spirit of God.
Understand your basic principle nature.

— Guru Amar Das, *Siri Guru Granth Sahib*,
page 441, line 3, as translated by Yogi Bhajan

If your nature, as a human, is angelic, God will come through you in every aspect. When it is not, then you have to co-exist. And co-existence is interdependent. It's mutual. But when you individually live in your ego, then it is barbaric. It is animal, and it has no redemption.

This principle of life that I am explaining to you is the law of the nature of the journey of the soul. Come with me. Let us walk. Let us carry this banner. Let us fly it high. Let us shed the light. Let us show the path. Let us consume ourselves for others. Let us carry others. Let us carry our children, carry ourselves and the child in us to that destiny that is marked on our forehead by the one self-hand of God almighty Himself.

That realization opens the Third Eye.

When a person realizes the Third Eye, this is the sight he sees—that the hand of God has written the destiny on the forehead of the person by itself, "by the Will of God." Then personal will goes away, ill will goes away, ego goes away and everything is Amigos; we live in a deep friendship with our soul, the spirit, our angelic nature, our divinity, our dignity, our grace and thus we achieve victory when we are alive and hereafter.

Then we are entitled to say, "*Wahe Guru Ji Ka Khalsa, Wahe Guru Ji Ki Fateh*." And I say to you all, "*Wahe Guru Ji Ka Khalsa, Wahe Guru Ji Ki Fateh*."

WHAT IS WAHE GURU?

1. Knowledge, talent and the secrets of success are in consistent pursuit.
2. Satisfaction, friendship and prosperity are in instant communication.
3. Every client is a super friend.
4. Every trade is a super opportunity.
5. Every smile is a direct achievement.
6. Every frown is a new loss.
7. Every hanky-panky is a loss of trust.
8. Every lie is a loss of face.
9. Every moment without understanding is a misunderstanding.
10. The power of victory is in strategy and action with a complete brief; result with complete assessment; recharge and attack again.
11. Every action must have cover and reinforcement.
12. Understand—then stand under.
13. If you want to get together, gather yourself first and then get together.
14. What we are, is what we do to others.
15. If we do not inspire others, we are depressed always.
16. If we do not love others, we practice self-hatred.
17. Any mistake takes away our prosperity.
18. Any loss is a challenge to prepare better.
19. Any tragedy is a challenge to wisdom.
20. Any treachery is a challenge to intelligence.
21. Any grief is to conquer the self.
22. This is all Wahe Guru.

© The Teachings of Yogi Bhajan,
September 11, 1996

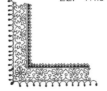

CHAPTER FIFTEEN

PREPARE YOURSELF TO SERVE THE AGE OF AQUARIUS

Life is based on touch. We touch each other with our eyes. We touch each other with our ears. We touch each other with songs and words. We touch physically. We touch to kill. We touch to give birth. If you look at the whole spectrum of life, it's nothing but touch. And if you want to know the Master's touch, then you should live by these words of Nanak.

ਆਦਿ ਸਚੁ ਜੁਗਾਦਿ ਸਚੁ ॥
ਹੈ ਭੀ ਸਚੁ ਨਾਨਕ ਹੋਸੀ ਭੀ ਸਚੁ ॥੧॥

Aad sach jugaad sach.
Hai bhee sach Naanak hosee bhee sach.

The world in the beginning was true, world throughout time is true, world now is true,
Nanak says this shall always be true.

— Guru Nanak, *Japji Sahib*, from the *Mul Mantra,*
as translated by Yogi Bhajan

That's the definition of touch. And that definition should become your touch. Nothing less than that will work. I am not teaching you philosophy or religion. I am teaching you reality. This is how you will enter the Age of Aquarius as leaders—rich, happy, healthy, creative, conscious, trustworthy and worthy.

Normally, you live by your own words. You live by your emotions; you live by your feelings; you live by your fantasies; you live by your desires; you live by the environments. You live by the call of your national emergencies, personal emergencies, cultural emergencies and other emergencies. You have a million things with which you divide yourself. But there is one thing that can fundamentally guide you to the height. Then nobody can touch you. And that height is,

ਆਦਿ ਸਚੁ ਜੁਗਾਦਿ ਸਚੁ ॥
ਹੈ ਭੀ ਸਚੁ ਨਾਨਕ ਹੋਸੀ ਭੀ ਸਚੁ ॥੧॥

Aad sach jugaad sach.
Hai bhee sach Naanak hosee bhee sach.

— Guru Nanak, *Japji Sahib*,
from the Mul Mantra

ਇਹੁ ਜਗੁ ਸਚੈ ਕੀ ਹੈ ਕੋਠੜੀ ਸਚੇ ਕਾ ਵਿਚਿ ਵਾਸੁ ॥

Ih jag sachai kee hai koth-rhee sachay kaa vich vaas.

This world is the house of truth and truth prevails

— Guru Angad, *Siri Guru Granth Sahib*,
page 463, line 13, as translated by Yogi Bhajan

It does not say "my" truth or "your" truth, "personal" truth or "impersonal" truth. Because your father didn't teach you right, therefore every man is a bastard. Because your mother didn't teach you right, therefore every woman is a bitch. No. That way of thinking is insanity. It's called qualified, determined, subverted insanity. That's the name in psychology for this. You cannot be you if you are caught in the past. If you have a past, you have no future. It's so funny how criminal you are.

When you drag your past into your future, first you have to bring in today. When you bring the past into today, then today—that precious time of life—is over. It's wasted. Then you have to drag that past from today into tomorrow, which has not yet come. So I don't think anybody is your enemy. You are your own enemy.

You have energy. Normally, people live on thirty percent of their personal energy. Seventy percent, they drag through their life. That's a lot of punishment. And then, we say we are spiritual. Then there's religion. Then God knows what. And what for? Why is there religion? Why is there a God when God made you in His own image, and created you in His own life span, and gave you destiny and distance. Why? Why?

Some boy was telling me, "I have meditated for twenty hours."

I said, "What for?" I was surprised. "In twenty hours, what did you do?"

He said, "I sat and did this kriya of yours for twenty hours."

"Twenty hours for what? Are you insane? I mean, if you are insane, you can meditate."

> *Life is a working meditation.*
> *A Master moves with*
> *mastery of meditation in*
> *every field of life.*
> *That's a Master.*

Life is a working meditation. A Master moves with mastery of meditation in every field of life. That's a Master. His majesty can be felt and seen without him uttering a word. You will have weight. Your personality will have weight. This is the simple formula. Learn it from me.

People will call you names and blame you. They'll go after you like hell.

At night, if you light a candle, by the morning, you will have two or three hundred dead moths. Which ones escaped? We don't know. What is their fight against? Their fight is against the light. If the candle is not lit, they are not going to come. And if, in life, you are not willing to take that challenge, then you are never ever going to be enlightened. It doesn't matter what you follow, who you follow, what you did, how many books you can cram, how many theories you have, how many certificates you have. As a human, without the challenge you are zero.

Human. Hue means light. Mann means mental. To me, now, you are a mental light. And you don't expect the moths to come near? That is a wrong concept of living.

The question is not whether the girl loves you. The question is, do you have control over yourself? If somebody loves you, do not love them if you cannot carry them. Don't betray people. Don't leave them. Be nice.

Touch a person, hold a person and then carry a person. You can't drag anybody. You can't lean on anybody. You can't do all those things where you can go wrong. Carry them, simply and truthfully. And what are the words that dignify the carrying?

Can you repeat after me? "I am with you." That's all. One line. "I am with you."

You know what I do when people shit at me? When they do, I sit there. It lasts from fifteen to forty-five minutes, depending on the capacity of the person. And you know what I say? "I am with you, don't worry. Nothing is going to happen. Go home, enjoy life." That's all.

You ask me why? The psychosomatic frequency in the molecule into the mega form can be changed into alpha, beta and theta, in the simple sense of the voice. That's a law nature must obey. It's not something people understand in a subtle way. But that's what the power is. That is the power of the word. Nobody can beat it. But you have to say, "I am with you."

The most veteran, courageous and pious act of a human is to be with another human. Because we are like stars in the sky, born at one time and space, to be ourselves. Everybody is our coherent neighbor. All we have to do is say, "I am with you."

When you start being one with everybody, then you are actually with God, because if you cannot see God in all, you cannot see God at all.

Let me give you an example. I received a telephone call and the person thought that since he has only been in 3HO for three months, what could he do to help someone else? The other person was going through changes. I told him, "Don't you worry. Just touch him, sit calmly and see what happens."

He said, "Should I do some mantra? Should I do a posture?"

"Just sit down with him and hold him. Touch him. He will be fine. If he is not fine in ten minutes, call me."

No phone call came after ten minutes, fifteen minutes, half an hour, or one hour. Finally the telephone rang. I understood and said, "Hey how is he?"

He said, "I don't know. He made me meditate."

"That guy who was so upset made you meditate?"

"Yes. It was so beautiful. I was in bliss. I was in ecstasy."

You see how helping others can work?

Do not misunderstand Guru Nanak. The whole life of Nanak is to help others. He walked, he talked, he visited places, he undertook impossible journeys, he started young. From the very first day, his job was to help others.

Symbolically, when you help others, Nanak comes in you. Don't call on him. He will be there. That is a personified prophecy. "If you walk one foot towards me I shall walk one thousand steps towards you." So technically speaking, it is not difficult. Understand Nanak once and for all. Forget who you are and help others. Nanak will take care of it in your life, in your family life, in your surroundings, in anything.

But one thing you have to do: forget yourself. I forgot, myself, that I am very, very sick. But see, I am on time and I am fine. Who is fine in me? Not me. Not at all. It's the same spirit of Nanak. Simply, I may have to lie about it. I recognize it and you don't. Sometimes, that's the difference. If you see only one word and understand the meaning of it, *Ang Sang Wahe Guru,* you don't have to learn anything else. I tell you this from my experience. Nanak shall come through and Guru Ram Das is nothing but a living miracle.

How beautiful will you be in the memory of another person if your very touch or presence or your few words can miraculously take care of the other person? Will he ever forget you? What I am saying is that for three thousand years, mankind has been taught that they are sinners, they are wrong, they are this, they are evil. That's one part.

The second part is that they need heaven. We need to have a comfortable time now. Heaven after death and this thing after that thing—you don't need that. All you need to do is to forget who you are and help another person. Reach out. This is life. "Hail Guru Ram Das and heal the world." And remember when you heal somebody's problem, your problem will disappear right under your own presence. You will love it. My problem, your problem, our problems are only there when we are not taking care of others. Do you understand? Marriages break, children go astray, neighbors fight. It doesn't mean anything. The Age of Aquarius is taking care of others.

You are you. You are within your God. But when you deal outside, touch everybody with the longing of the soul. That enriches your soul. That's why Guru Nanak gave only one order. *Jap.* It means means repeat. There is one commandment. Very martial. *Jap.* And what do we repeat?

ਆਦਿ ਸਚੁ ਜੁਗਾਦਿ ਸਚੁ ॥
ਹੈ ਭੀ ਸਚੁ ਨਾਨਕ ਹੋਸੀ ਭੀ ਸਚੁ ॥੧॥

Aad sach, jugad sach, hai bhee sach, Naanak hosee bhee sach.

In the beginning it is true, through the time it is true, now is true,
and Nanak says it shall always be true.

If you just believe that, then Mother Nature will give you a place where your legacy will live forever.

The human race without grace shall not enter the Age of Aquarius. I am not sure that you will not experience tragedy after tragedy, because the psychosomatics of the earth axle, the magnetic field and the flare of the sun into the creativity and reflection of the moon have already changed.

Soon you might ask for a day of atonement and want to lie down in a coffin, so you can close your eyes. That's how bad it can be in the years before the Aquarian Age begins. These years are the years of challenge. And what is the challenge? You must come to embrace the truth. You must come and experience the truth. You must come and be the truth. Like *Aad sach* it was. So you are *Aad sach*.

Keep your *sadhana*—regardless of how you feel about it. Do not feel somebody is better or worse than you. If you continue your *sadhana*, the end result will be that you will be needed by the Age of Aquarius. Try to understand how lucky you are. We are going through a change of age and we are participating in it. It is not that a huge disaster should happen and only then will people see the age is changing. If you look at the evening news you will find that disasters are happening everywhere. But you are changing. You are changing to challenge the ultimate challenge—to help humanity through it.

Once I was teaching in Berkeley University and a guy about six foot and some inches tall, took a knife and started dancing over me. Everybody wanted to eat him alive and show him how good his meat was, but, I said, "No." I kept sitting, and we kept talking. In the end, he got tired. He sat down and he did the class. After the class was finished, some people wanted to teach him a lesson but I said, "No. Leave him alone."

So he came to me and he said, "Master, I have a question."

I said, "Go ahead."

"I was dancing with a naked knife over you. Why do you think I wouldn't stab you?"

"Because that doesn't work. If you have to stab me, you'd stab me. You took so much time dancing. You didn't have the energy to stab. And why should you stab me?"

"I would have liked to stab you."

"Try it now. Now that we are on a one-on-one basis."

"Why are you so sure?"

"I am a trained commando. Before you even think of stabbing me, I'll teach you a lesson. I'll take each of your ribs and put them in your hands before you close your eyes. Do you want to see that?"

"No, no, no, no, no. I was joking. It's okay."

"If you are joking, then I am joking, too. Then we have nothing to fight about. We have nothing to be angry about."

And then he said, "But I did disturb your class."

I said, "No, you brought out the best in me. Tomorrow, when I go to teach class, there will be double the number of students. Don't worry. It's good P.R."

And it was true. That's why I say—patience pays. Patience pays.

When you lose your patience and you don't have patience, then you don't have yourself. It's a most cowardly act. When you lash out and flash out and do all that mischief, you are cheap and you are a creep. It's not you. Hold your ground and behold. Every day is yours and yours alone. It is not anybody else's. Behold, the breath of life is yours. This life is yours. You are yours. How many of you are yours? How many have given themselves to themselves? What kind of lover are you? What an idiotic thing to do—to love everybody, but not yourself.

"Hi, honey. Where are we going to eat?"

Have you ever said to yourself, "Hey body, where are we going to exercise, eat and be nice?"

You think it is insanity to talk to your Self—which is so powerful in you and living and beautiful and gorgeous? How can an empty glass take away the thirst of anybody? How can a man who is empty, unloving and absolutely uncaring, care for anybody, except the emotions? You find a problem—that you are lonely. You are just creating animosity with your own self because you are *never* lonely. You have God, you have *Guru*, you have your Self, three. You are number four. How lonely can you be? But you've said you are lonely. So within your own cycle and circle, you have daydreams, you have nightmares, you have fantasies and you have commotions.

That is what comes to experience a Master's touch. And when you touch a Master, you become the Master.

Paaras is the philosopher's stone. When it touches anything, it makes it gold. They say a stone went to paaras and became gold. *Mitay pavan.* Then all the cycles, the circle of life is finished. We have to do that now.

The world is going to hold onto us. If we will not prepare ourselves to face it, we may become failures.

People say to us, "You look beautiful. Help me." They don't want to tell you a story, they don't want to take time.

You have to help them. You can't hide under this nonsense, under your neurotic life. "Oh, I am an attorney. I am a doctor. I am an executive. I am successful." People won't care who you are. People will mob you. They will ask for help. They will like your energy; they will want the touch. If you know how to touch the heart, you will be great. You will be positive. What more I can tell you? It's on us. It is coming. We have prepared ourselves for thirty years. That's why we have not done too much PR or too much drama, too much this or too much that. No, no, no, no, no. If you know God and *Guru* and you do not know evil and the devil, then you know nothing. Things are always in twos. The coin has both sides. One side is the state, the other is the kingly head. Metal is the same. You have to know what is wrong and what is right. Then you can find what is wrong and then you can substitute with right. Otherwise there is no need to prostitute your life. Nobody can tell you what to do. You have to go sincerely inside your psyche and say, "I am radiant. I am a reality. I have my own reverence."

Let people know you are a graceful reality, with reverence of courage. You have to protect your own reverence. Nobody can protect it for you.

Now I have done my job. I am on my way out. I have come, lived my promise to create teachers. Teachers are those who will practice the teachings in reality. If there is no experience, get the experience. The time has come now that you should become teachers and cover me. I have covered you. I did not come here for students. I came here to create teachers. I have done my job silently, in shame, in pain, in slander, in praise, in appreciation, in service and in disaster. It didn't matter because the pair of opposites does not affect a yogi. I have given you all that you need. For your sake, practice it and experience it so you can share with people who will fall on you like hordes.

Thank you very much. May you all be blessed, blessed, blessed and may Guru Ram Das bless you forever. This is the time for you to declare yourself. You are teachers and even if you have been the most lazy, lousy, bedridden, nonsense, come out and just touch people. Leave the rest to God. Be kind, compassionate and caring. And just touch. Everybody has obnoxiousness and passion and everybody has compassion and grace equal to it. So, there is no dearth of natural faculties to be positive. We are going to play the biggest show on this earth, the greatest show of all time, as Aquarian teachers and that's what you all are.

Kindness knows no defeat. Caring has no end. And touching a person's heart is the only language God knows. I hope God and *Guru* will bless you throughout this time, here and hereafter.

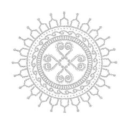

Kriyas, Meditations
and Shabad Practices

Before You Begin

Beginning Your Practice—Tuning In

The practice of Kundalini Yoga as taught by Yogi Bhajan® always begins by tuning in. This simple practice of chanting *Ong Namo Guru Dev Namo* 3 to 5 times, aligns your mind, your spirit and your body to become alert and assert your will so that your practice will fulfill its intention. It's a simple bowing to your Higher Self and an alignment with the teacher within. The mantra is simple but it links you to a Golden Chain of teachers, an entire body of consciousness that guides and protects your practice: Ong Namo Guroo Dayv Namo, which means, "I bow to the Infinite, I bow to the Teacher within."

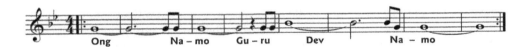

How to End

Another tradition within Kundalini Yoga as taught by Yogi Bhajan® is a simple blessing known as *The Long Time Sun Shine* song. Sung or simply recited at the end of your practice, it allows you to dedicate your practice to all those who've preserved and delivered these teachings so that you might have the experience of your Self. It is a simple prayer to bless yourself and others, which completes the practice and allows your entire discipline to become a prayer, in service to the good of all.

May the long time sun
shine upon you

All love surround you

And the pure light
within you

Guide your way on.

Sat Nam.

Other Tips for a Successful Experience

Prepare for your practice by lining up all the elements that will elevate your experience: natural fiber clothing and head covering (cotton or linen), preferably white to increase your auric body; natural fiber mat, either cotton or wool; traditionally a sheep skin or other animal skin is used. If you have to use a rubber or petroleum-based mat, cover the surface with a cotton or wool blanket to protect and support your electromagnetic field. Clean air and fresh water also help support your practice. These are ideal conditions, but in today's society, taking the time to do a simple *pranayam* at your desk or spine flex in the conference room or chanting in the kitchen while your child takes a nap can go a long way toward making your day more productive and relaxing.

Practice in Community

Kundalini Yoga cultivates group consciousness, because group consciousness is the first step toward universal consciousness, which is the goal: transcend the ego and merge with Infinity. Therefore, find a teacher in your area. Studying the science of Kundalini Yoga with a KRI certified teacher will enhance your experience and deepen your understanding of kriya, mantra, breath and posture. If there isn't a teacher in your area, consider becoming a teacher yourself. See our resources page for more information.

Find a group to practice sadhana (daily spiritual routine) with, or establish a group sadhana yourself—in your home or community center. The Aquarian Sadhana[45] was given by Yogi Bhajan to ground our practice now and into the Aquarian Age. Practicing with others increases the effects of sadhana exponentially. You heal others and others, in turn, heal you. Begin Full Moon gatherings, bringing together women from all areas of life to celebrate, meditate and heal one another. Start a Peanut Hour with mothers in your neighborhood, or friends in your community, church, or workplace. Come together as women and share your strength, ask for help when you need it and laugh together as you participate in this game of life.

Breath & Bandhas[46]

Long Deep Breath

To take a full yogic breath, inhale by first relaxing the abdomen and allow it to expand. Next expand the chest and finally the collarbones. As you exhale let the collarbones and chest relax first, then pull the abdomen in completely.

The diaphragm drops down to expand the lungs on the inhale and contracts up to expel the air on the exhale.

As you inhale feel the back area of the lower ribs relax and expand. On the exhale be sure to keep the spine erect and steady.

---

[45] See *Kundalini Yoga Sadhana Guidelines, 2nd Edition,* available from the Kundalini Research Institute, for more information about creating your own sadhana and guidelines for practicing the Aquarian Sadhana.
[46] from *Kundalini Yoga Sadhana Guidelines, 2nd Edition.*

Breath of Fire

This breath is used consistently throughout Kundalini Yoga kriyas. It is very important that Breath of Fire be practiced and mastered. In Breath of Fire, the focus of the energy is at the navel point. The breath is fairly rapid (approximately 2 breaths per second), continuous and powerful with no pause between the inhale and exhale. This is a balanced breath with no emphasis on either the exhale or the inhale, but rather equal power given to both.

Breath of Fire is a cleansing breath, which renews the blood and releases old toxins from the lungs, mucous lining, blood vessels and cells. It is a powerful way to adjust your autonomic nervous system and get rid of stress. Regular practice expands the lungs quickly.

Cannon Breath

Cannon Breath is a powerful inhalation and exhalation through the mouth, with a slight pause between the inhalation and exhalation. Very cleansing, this breath is invigorating, energizing and rejuvenating.

To consolidate the energy at the end of a kriya, many will call for a Cannon Fire exhale, which means you suspend the breath on the inhale and then use a single strong exhale through the mouth like a cannon.

Bandhas

Bandhas, or locks, are used frequently in Kundalini Yoga. Combinations of muscle contractions, each lock has the function of changing blood circulation, nerve pressure and the flow of cerebral spinal fluid. They also direct the flow of psychic energy or *prana*, into the main energy channels that relate to raising the kundalini energy. They concentrate the body's energy for use in consciousness and self-healing. There are three important locks: *jalandhar bandh, uddiyana bandh* and *mulbandh*. When all three locks are applied simultaneously, it is called *mahabandh*, the Great Lock.

Jalandhar Bandh or *Neck Lock*

The most basic lock used in Kundalini Yoga is *jalandhar bandh*, the neck lock. This lock is practiced by gently stretching the back of the neck straight and pulling the chin toward the back of the neck. Lift the chest and sternum and keep the muscles of the neck and throat and face relaxed.

Uddiyana Bandh or *Diaphragm Lock*

Applied by lifting the diaphragm up high into the thorax and pulling the upper abdominal muscles back toward the spine, *uddiyana bandh* gently massages the intestines and the heart muscle. The spine should be straight and it is most often applied on the exhale.

Applied forcefully on the inhale, it can create pressure in the eyes and the heart.

Mulbandh or Root Lock

The Root Lock is the most commonly applied lock but also the most complex. It coordinates and combines the energy of the rectum, sex organs, and navel point.

Mul is the root, base, or source. The first part of the *mulbandh* is to contract the anal sphincter and draw it in and up as if trying to hold back a bowel movement. Then draw up the sex organ so the urethral tract is contracted. Finally, pull in the navel point by drawing back the lower abdomen towards the spine so the rectum and sex organs are drawn up toward the navel point.

Pronunciation Guide

This simple guide to the vowel sounds in transliteration is for your convenience. More commonly used words are often spelled traditionally, for example, Nanak, Sat Nam, Wahe Guru, or pranayam, even though you'll often see them written Naanak, Sat Naam, Whaa-hay Guroo, and praanayaam, in order to clarify the pronunciation, especially in mantras.

Gurbani is a very sophisticated sound system, and there are many other guidelines regarding consonant sounds and other rules of the language that are best conveyed through a direct student-teacher relationship. Further guidelines regarding pronunciation are available at www.kundaliniresearchinstitute.org.

a	hut
aa	mom
u	put, soot
oo	pool
i	fin
ee	feet
ai	let
ay	hay, rain
r	flick tongue on upper palate

A Note to the Practitioner

All comments found within the kriyas and meditations are from Yogi Bhajan unless otherwise indicated.

PART ONE

EXPANDING YOUR IDENTITY

BRING PROSPERITY TO YOUR LIFE
December 26, 1997

PART ONE

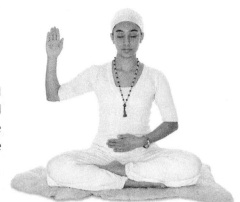

POSTURE: Sit in Easy Pose.

MUDRA: Raise the forearm of the right hand as if you were taking an oath. The right hand faces forward at the level of the ear. With the left hand, gently cover the Navel Point. Become a statue.

EYES: The eyes are closed.

BREATH AND FOCUS: Slowly allow your breath to become a little longer, deeper and cooler. By allowing this to happen, you will change your metabolism and your nervous system, and you will be totally different. Focus on the breath—take it as deep as you can. Don't move except to breathe long and deep. Take the pranic energy down to the last cell of the lungs.

TO END: Relax out of the posture.

TIME: 8 minutes

COMMENTS: Just be you. Be you—calm, quiet, graceful, clean, gracious and self-serving. Be you and be selfish for your own purity and piety. All we want is the result. We're not trying to find diamonds or gold. We are finding something more precious than that—Self. Find your Self. Find "me" within me.

The Navel Point is the one point in the body that is a point of purity. You survived in your mother because of that point. Here, you touch that point with the left hand and extend the fingers of the right hand up like antenna—they are enough to get all the energy of Jupiter, Saturn, Sun and Mercury. This posture, in combination with your id, the thumb, will make the connection so that the heavens and the earth—the heavenly father and Mother Nature—are in combination. Together they are willing to purify you if you ask for it. Technically speaking, the calmer you sit, the deeper you breathe, the more you will experience a change you have never felt before.

(continued on next page)

Think only of your Self and the breath. Let the breath of life enrich you. Let it give you a place within yourself where you can see your God—which is keeping you alive. Your soul needs food. It is hungry and it needs you to feed it. The soul's diet is the *prana* that comes through the air to enrich you from the inside out. Reach for a moment of happiness. Happiness is when you happily do something. Otherwise, life is a painful curse.

PART TWO

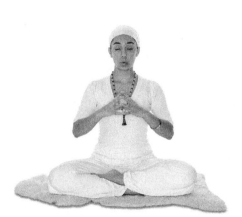

POSTURE: Continue sitting in Easy Pose.

MUDRA: Bring the hands to the level of the Heart Center. Press the thumb tips and fingertips together, keeping the palms apart. Spread the fingers wide apart and point the thumbs toward the sternum.

BREATH: Whistle with the Ardas Bhaee chant.

TIME: 4 ½ minutes

TO END: Inhale deeply and suspend the breath for **15 seconds**. Meditate on the thought that you are pure; you are perfect; you are the will of God; you are divine. Exhale. Inhale again and suspend the breath for **15 seconds** and create that image of yourself. Exhale. Inhale a third time and hold the breath tight for **15 seconds**. Imagine you are a very, very pure person. Purity, piety, grace, bliss—include them all. Exhale.

PART THREE

POSTURE: Immediately extend the arms straight out to each side at shoulder level, parallel to the ground, with the right palm facing up and the left palm facing down. Keep the arms and hands straight. You may feel a twist in the right elbow. This is a healing posture to be done very exactly.

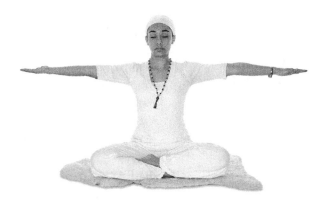

BREATH: Inhale deeply and suspend the breath for **25 seconds**. Close your eyes and feel the heavens and earth are joining within you. Concentrate on your left side and your right side uniting in oneness. Keep the hands straight like an arrow. Cannon fire out through the mouth. Inhale deeply again. Hold tight for **25 seconds**. Give yourself a chance to heal yourself totally—in balance with the Universe. In the divine kingdom, be divine. Cannon fire out. Inhale again. Hold tight for **25 seconds**. With great kindness to your Self consider, "It is me and my purity that will give me health, wealth and happiness." Call on it. Exhale and relax.

TIME: 2 minutes

COMMENTS: Yogi Bhajan suggested that you could practice this kriya for up to 62 minutes by dividing the time equally among the three parts. If you extend the times, don't extend them proportionately, practice each part equally.

You have unlimited reserve energy. When you invoke your energy, there's nothing that is small in you and all the environments start flying towards you. It's beautiful. It is a way of life.

Become a human. Find your Self within yourself and then see what comes to you. That's my challenge to you. Just be yourself with everybody. Say, "Hello. Thank you. Can I do something for you?" That's all it is.

Let the Self Take Care of Things
November 10, 2001

Part One

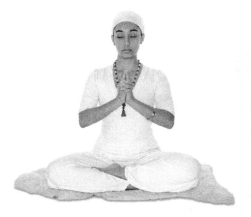

POSTURE: Sit straight in Easy Pose.

MUDRA: Hold your hands together in Sarab Gyan Mudra in front of the heart. Begin by interlacing the fingers, then extend the index fingers up, pressing the palms and index fingers very tightly together, thumbs crossed.

EYES: The eyes are closed.

BREATH: With Long Deep Breathing, meditate on your breath, inhaling and exhaling so deeply and completely that you can hear your own breath. Each breath should be a voluntary, mechanical breath. **11 minutes**.

Part Two

POSTURE: Sarab Gyan Mudra

BREATH: Do Long Deep Breathing in rhythm with the mantra, *Sat Narayan Wahe Guru Hari Narayan Sat Nam* as recorded by Mata Mandir Singh, inhaling during one complete sound cycle (2 repetitions of the mantra, about 20 seconds) and exhaling during one complete sound cycle (2 repetitions of the mantra). **11 minutes.**

PART THREE

POSTURE & MUDRA: Same as Parts One & Two

BREATH: Do a powerful Breath of Fire. Continue for **3 minutes**, doing your best during the last minute.

TO END: Inhale deeply, suspend the breath and exhale. Repeat 1 more time. Relax.

COMMENTS: In this meditation you must concentrate on your breath. The moment it starts affecting your metabolism, you will start to feel light, then knowledgeable and then your sense of security will start increasing. You should breathe, not your body! Meditate deeply on your breath and increase your self-control. If the Self starts working, it will take care of things. There is nothing more important than your Self. You have to change the frequency of your psyche and change the degree of your expansion of consciousness. When you understand and practice compassion, what you want can come to you 100 times! But you have to act responsibly and consciously. Work. Be. Have more success in business and make more money so that you can help more people. Give them peace, tranquility and grace. Trust your Self so people can trust you.

SUBAGH KRIYA

June 21, 1996

Each exercise in this five-part kriya must be done for the same length of time, either **3 minutes** each or **11 minutes** each.

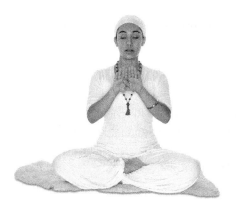

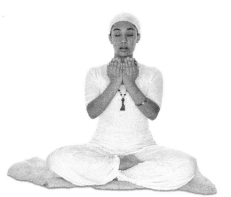

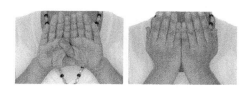

PART ONE

POSITION: Sit in Easy Pose with a light *Jalandhar Bandh*.

MUDRA: Bend the elbows, angling the forearms up and outward with the fingers at the level of the throat. Begin with the palms facing down.

Alternately hit the sides of the hands together timed with the mantra below. When the hands hit facing down, the sides of the Jupiter (index) fingers touch and the thumbs cross below the hands, with the right thumb under the left. Yogi Bhajan said that crossing the thumbs in this way is the key to the meditation. When the hands hit facing up, the Mercury (pinkie) fingers and the Moon Mounds (located on the bottom of the palms) hit.

EYE FOCUS: The eyes are 1/10th open. Focus at the tip of the nose.

MANTRA: Chant the mantra *HAR* with the tip of your tongue as you alternately strike the Jupiter area (palms facing down) and the Moon area (palms facing up). Pull the navel with each *HAR*. This meditation was taught to the rhythm of *Tantric Har* by Simran Kaur.

TIME: 3-11 minutes.

COMMENTS: You should not do this exercise more than 3 minutes when you are working during the day, or you will become too rich. I am not joking. Doing it for 11 minutes a day is more than enough. Doing it too much will be greed. It stimulates the mind, the Moon Center and Jupiter. When Jupiter and the moon come together, there is no way in the world you will not make wealth.

NOTE: Part One can be done on its own for prosperity.

PART TWO

POSITION: Stretch your arms out to the sides and raise them up to a V shape at a 60-degree angle. Face the palms forward and spread your fingers wide, making them stiff. On the exhale, cross your arms in front of your face, left arm in front of the right. Inhale and return your arms out to the V shape. Continue crossing the arms, keeping the elbows straight and the fingers open and stiff, alternating the position of the arms as they cross.

EYES: The eyes remain closed.

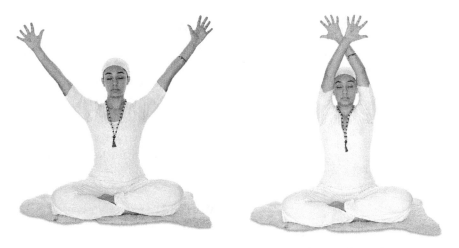

MANTRA: Move the arms in rhythm with the *Tantric Har*, but do not chant this time.

(continued on next page)

PART THREE

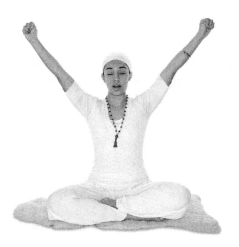

POSITION: Keep your arms extended at 60 degrees. With your fingers, make a fist around your thumb, squeezing your thumb tightly as if you are trying to squeeze all the blood out of it. Move your arms in small backward circles as you continue squeezing your thumb. Keep the arms stretched with the elbows straight. Move so powerfully that your entire spine shakes— you may even lift slightly up off the ground.

MANTRA: Chant the mantra *GOD* powerfully from your navel. One backward circle of the arms equals one repetition of *GOD*. The speed and rhythm of the chanting are the same as in the previous exercises.

PART FOUR

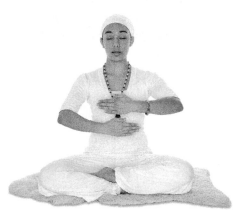

POSITION: Bend your arms so that your forearms are parallel to the floor and the palms face the body at the level of the diaphragm. One palm (it does not matter which) is closer to your body. To begin, the right hand moves up a few inches as the left hand moves down. The hands move alternately up and down between the Heart Center and Navel Center in a smooth motion to the rhythm of the mantra below.

MANTRA: As the hands move, chant *HAR HARAY HAREE, WHAA-HAY GUROO* in a deep monotone with one repetition of the mantra approximately every 4 seconds. Chant from your navel.

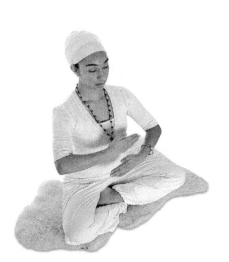

TIME: If you are practicing the exercises for **11 minutes** each, chant the mantra out loud for **6 minutes**, whisper it strongly for **3 minutes**

and then whistle it for **2 minutes**. If you are practicing the exercises for **3 minutes** each, chant the mantra out loud for **1 minute**, whisper it strongly for **1 minute**, and then whistle it for **1 minute**.

PART FIVE

POSITION: Bend the arms in front of the chest and rest the right forearm on the left forearm, palms facing down. Keep the spine straight and keep the arms steady and parallel to the ground; don't let them fall.

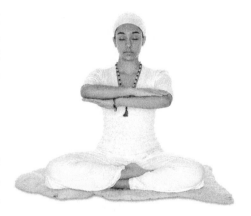

EYES: The eyes are closed.

BREATH: One-minute breath. Breathe slowly and deeply so that one breath takes a full minute. Breathing consciously, inhale for 20 seconds, hold for 20 seconds and exhale for 20 seconds.

COMMENTS: It's a complete set. This is all called Subagh Kriya. If God has written with His own hands that you shall live under misfortune, then by doing Subagh Kriya you can turn your misfortune into prosperity, fortune and good luck.

By tendency you are not very agreeable most of the time. You are more concerned with your scare tactics and insecurities than with your power to expand. I'm going to give you a very handy tool—one that you can use anywhere—and you'll become rich. I'm not going to give you printed money, but I will give you a tool for prosperity. I would like you to be your own judge and see how it works. There are a lot of things you can't do. You can't look unique. You can't look extraordinary. You don't want to be excellent because you are afraid of the responsibility. But if the psyche is corrected once in a while—for a few minutes here and a few minutes there—you will be surprised how much good you can do for yourself.

To become rich and prosperous with wealth and values, is to have the strength to come through. It means that the transmissions from your brain and the power of your intuition can immediately tell you what to do. You will be in a position to change gears smoothly. If you need to go in reverse, you can go in reverse. If you need to go forward, you'll go forward. This is a very old and simple system.

THREE-MINUTE HAR

POSITION: Sit in Easy Pose with a light Jalandhar Bandh.

MUDRA: Bend the elbows, angling the forearms up and outward with the fingers at the level of the throat. Begin with the palms facing down.

Alternately hit the sides of the hands together timed with the mantra below. When the hands hit facing down, the sides of the Jupiter (index) fingers touch and the thumbs cross below the hands, with the right thumb under the left. Yogi Bhajan said that crossing the thumbs in this way is the key to the meditation. When the hands hit facing up, the Mercury (pinkie) fingers and the Moon Mounds (located on the bottom of the palms) hit.

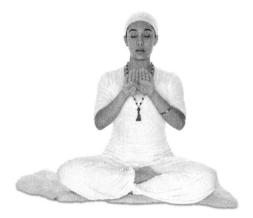

EYE FOCUS: The eyes are 1/10th open. Look at the tip of the nose.

MANTRA: Chant the mantra *HAR* with the tip of your tongue as you alternately strike the Jupiter area (palms facing down) and the Moon area (palms facing up). Pull the navel with each *HAR*. (This meditation was taught to the rhythm of *Tantric Har* by Simran Kaur.)

TIME: Continue for **3-11 minutes.**

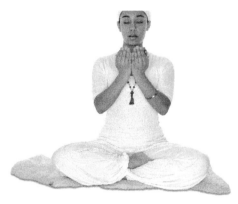

COMMENTS: You should not do this exercise more than 3 minutes when you are working during the day, or you will become too rich. I am not joking. Doing it for 11 minutes a day is more than enough. Doing it too much will be greed. It stimulates the mind, the Moon Center, and Jupiter. When Jupiter and the moon come together, there is no way in the world you will not make wealth.

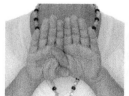
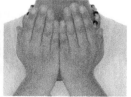

EXPERIENCE YOUR OWN SOUL BLESSING YOU WITH PROSPERITY

This meditation will elevate your energy so strongly that you can easily experience your own soul blessing you with prosperity.

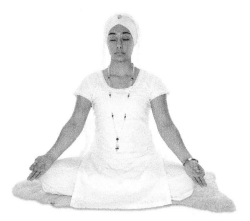

POSTURE: Sit in Easy Pose (or on a chair) with a straight spine.

MUDRA: Hands rest on knees in Gyan Mudra (index finger and thumb tip touching).

EYE FOCUS: The eyes are 1/10th open. Focus at the tip of the nose.

MANTRA: Repeat the entire mantra on a single breath in a relaxed monotone that varies in emphasis automatically as you proceed through the stages of the mantra.

HAR HAR HAR HAR, WHAA-HAY GUROO, SAT NAAM, HAR HAREE

The first part of the mantra, *HAR HAR HAR HAR*, is the beginning of your energetic journey. Place these sounds at the Third Chakra (Navel Point) to initiate the Kundalini energy. *HAR* means "God in creativity." Pull in the navel slightly with each repetition.

The second stage of the mantra is *WHAA-HAY GUROO*. Place this sound at the Heart Chakra, as you pull Diaphragm Lock, simultaneously pulling the Navel Point towards the spine. Hold these two locks fixed for the rest of the mantra.

The third stage is *SAT NAAM*. Project this sound from the Fifth Chakra at the throat. As you chant, gently apply Neck Lock.

The last part of the mantra is *HAR HAREE*. *HAR* is placed at the Sixth Chakra, and Haree goes through the top of the Seventh Chakra to Infinity. The eyes may automatically rise up a bit at this point.

Quickly inhale, bringing the cycle of energy and attention back to the Third Chakra, while relaxing the locks. Repeat the mantra again. Let yourself be drawn more and more deeply into this sound current.

TIME: Start with **11 minutes** and work up to **31 minutes**.

ICCHA KRIYA
April 14, 1992

NOTE: There are no breaks or pauses between the parts of this meditation.

PART ONE

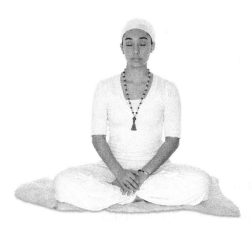

POSTURE: Come into Easy Pose. Sit in this relaxed posture, in tranquility and grace.

MUDRA: Place the hands in your lap, both palms facing down, right hand on top of the left, both palms facing down.

EYES: The eyes are closed.

FOCUS: Start thinking. Just think. And whatever you think, add, "What am I thinking?" It's simple and the oldest method of cross-reference thinking. The idea is to realize, "Oh, I am thinking. What am I thinking? I am thinking something. What is that something?" Then keep going. See where it takes you. As long as your right hand is over your left hand, it works. Keep thinking. Don't worry, and don't stop. Keep pursuing the thought. One thought will release another thought, then that thought will release another. See if you can stop somewhere. **3 minutes**.

PART TWO

Keep your eyes closed. Keep your posture with your hands on the lap. But take your tongue and begin to flick it like a snake, in and out. Keep thinking. Your tongue has nothing to do with you. The snake breathes and cools himself through the tongue. Similarly, your tongue will move. It's just not split, that's all. Keep thinking and pursue each thought. Once in a while, at your pleasure, flick your tongue like a snake. The tongue must leave your lips and show up in the air. Don't pull it all out—but extend it a little. **5 minutes**.

PART THREE

Continue as in Part Two. Listen to *Say Saraswati* by Nirinjan Kaur. **7 minutes**.

PART FOUR

Continue listening to the music as in Part Three. Now consciously think about your first fear, your primal fear. In this meditation, just concentrate on one primal fear. It's between you and you. No one else will know it. It's very important to keep your eyes closed while you are thinking about your fear. Under no circumstances should you open your eyes. **6 minutes.**

TO END: Inhale. Hold tight and move your body in complete circles, like a convulsion. **20 seconds**. Exhale.

Inhale again. Hold the breath and move all parts of the body very powerfully—to equalize the energy in every part of the body. **20 seconds**. All the organs need the benefits. Exhale.

Inhale again—deeply. Hold tight. This time, don't spare any part. Move everything—powerfully, strongly, tightly—holding the breath of life inside. You have to go through it for your own health and happiness. **20 seconds**. Exhale. Relax for a few minutes.

PART FIVE

Everything has come to a consolidated zero and now has to be moved. Put on some bhangara or other strong dance rhythms, and move the shoulders, heart, arms and rib cage in rhythm with the music. The rib cage is the main thing. If you can move your body vigorously in this, you can totally heal your physical self. **3 minutes**.

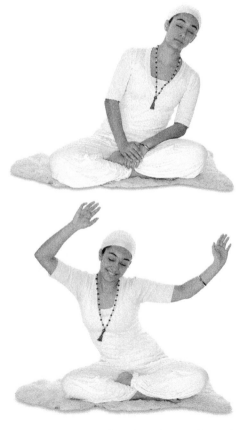

COMMENTS: There is a snake called *Iccha Naag*—it is always a cobra. *Iccha Naag* is a snake that only has to wish to have things magnetically come to him. What you are doing is called *Iccha Kriya*. You can magnetically get what you want.

You develop your psyche by your fears. Your fears are what limit you. They cut you out from the totality of life. This exercise is unique and very scientific. If you do it right technically, you will realize something you can't realize otherwise.

(continued on next page)

The scientific explanation is that your *shushmana*, or central nerve, is in the center of your tongue. When you pull on it by moving your tongue in and out, your thoughts come to a purification under its commanding will. If that is developed, you can get anything you want.

There are techniques like this—methodologies and formulas from wise elders—that can totally take you out of all kinds of dangers. It comes down to the basic truth that God is perfect, Omnipresent, Omniscient, whatever you want to call Him. He can't create anything incomplete. You are complete for the purposes of longitude and latitude, circumstances and confrontation.

SELF-CONTAINMENT AND EXPANSION

August 2, 2001

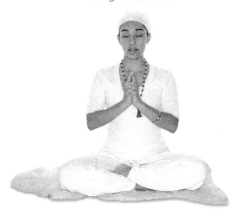

POSTURE: Sit straight in Easy Pose.

MUDRA: Hold your hands in Sarab Gyan Mudra in front of the Heart Center. Begin by interlacing the fingers, then extend the index fingers up, pressing the palms and index fingers very tightly together, thumbs crossed. The elbows are relaxed.

EYE FOCUS: The eyes are 1/10th open. Focus at the tip of the nose.

MANTRA: Chant the Ik Acharee Chand[47] shabad from the navel using the recording by Gurushabd Singh and Nirinjan Kaur.

Ajai Alai	Invincible, Indestructible
Abhai Abai	Fearless, Unchanging
Abhoo Ajoo	Unformed, Unborn
Anaas Akaas	Imperishable, Etheric
Aganj Abhanj	Unbreakable, Impenetrable
Alakh Abhakh	Unseen, Unaffected
Akaal Dyaal	Undying, Merciful
Alaykh Abhaykh	Indescribable, Uncostumed
Anaam Akaam	Nameless, Desireless
Agaahaa Adhaahaa	Unfathomable, Incorruptible
Anaathay Paramaathay	Unmastered, Destroyer
Ajonee Amonee	Beyond birth, Beyond silence
Na Raagay Na Rangay	Beyond love, Beyond color
Na Roopay Na Raykhay	Beyond form, Beyond shape
Akaramang Abharamang	Beyond karma, Beyond doubt
Aganjay Alaykhay	Unconquerable, Indescribable

---

[47] The ***Ik Acharee Chand*** shabad is from ***Jaap Sahib***, by Guru Gobind Singh.

(continued on next page)

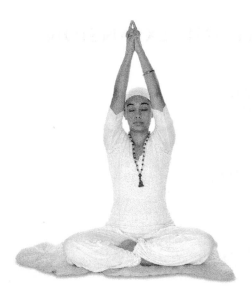

TIME: 31 minutes.

TO END: Inhale deeply and hold the breath while stretching the arms up and maintaining the hand position. Continuing to stretch, exhale. Repeat 2 times and relax.

COMMENTS BY DR. GURUCHARAN SINGH KHALSA

This mudra brings a sense of self-containment because the hands are interlocked at the Heart Chakra. It evokes the expansion from the planet Jupiter, the index finger. When you practice this posture with this most exalted mantra and experience the ownership of a more expanded, prosperous existence, prosperity will surely come.

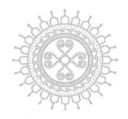

PART TWO

CLEARING THE BLOCKS

GET RID OF YOUR "COULDN'T"

September 4, 2001

POSTURE: Sit straight and tall in Easy Pose, as if you were the Lord Buddha.

MUDRA: Cross the middle fingers over the backs of the index fingers, locking the other two fingers down with the thumbs. Bend the elbows and bring the mudra up to ear level.

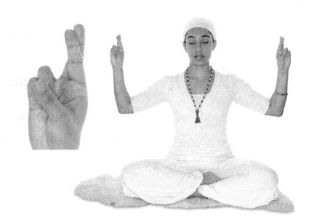

EYES: The eyes are closed.

MANTRA: Chant *Har* from the navel to the rhythm of *Tantric Har* by Simran Kaur and Guru Prem Singh. Be constant and consistent.

TIME: 11 minutes.

TO END: Inhale deeply, hold. Let the breath and the mantra multiply into your being. Exhale. Repeat. Then one more time inhale deeply and powerfully, hold, and pull the navel in. Exhale and relax.

COMMENTS: Do you remember when you wanted to come to class and you said, "I couldn't"? Do you remember when you wanted to get up in the morning and be with your God and instead said, "I couldn't"? Do you remember when you wanted to love and be with somebody and decided, "I couldn't"? All the problems on this planet come from this "couldn't." It gives us a slip from our dharma, from our destiny. We need to make our will so clean, clear and positive that "couldn't" does not touch our shores. Kundalini Yoga takes away our "couldn't" and gives us our excellence.

Every sequence has a consequence. When we start a sequence, the consequence will be there. If you do not want consequences, do not start the sequence. Have that control! Control your "couldn't!"

Practicing a kriya with a mantra like this one gives you a rhythm. When your life is subject to rhythm, your "couldn't" goes away.

DEVELOP YOUR CROSS-REFERENCE
October 16, 1993

PART ONE

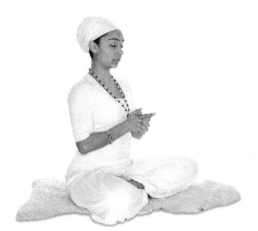

POSTURE: Come into Easy Pose.

MUDRA: Relax the elbows at your sides with the forearms touching the body. Interlace your fingers and thumbs except for the Jupiter (index) fingers at the solar plexus. The Jupiter fingers are extended together, pointing out from the body. Keep your posture absolutely solid and straight.

MENTAL FOCUS: Concentrate on your Jupiter finger and mentally project one phrase: "Proper, power and prosperity." Think prosperity, feel prosperity and meditate on prosperity. Get into a solid state and cut out all other thoughts.

EYE FOCUS: The eyes are closed, looking at the chin through the closed eyes.

MUSIC: Listen, without chanting, to *Prosperity* by Nirinjan Kaur. The music is to support the meditative concentration.

I know Thou Thee
Whaa-hay
Guroo Jee.
Give my day prosperity.
Reality, prosperity and ecstasy.

TIME: 1 minute to get into a solid state with "Proper, power and prosperity." **11 minutes** silently meditating with the musical affirmation. **12 minutes** total.

TO END: Inhale deeply, hold tight and keep meditating. Circulate your breath like an energy field. Put your disappointments in it. **20 seconds**. Let it go. Inhale deeply again and let the breath circulate in you, gathering all your disappointments and disillusions. **20 seconds**. And let it go. Inhale deeply and suspend the breath. **10 seconds**. Relax.

PART TWO

EYES: The eyes are closed.

MUDRA: The arms are parallel to the floor, in front of and not touching the body, elbows out, at the heart level. The left hand is palm down in a fist with the Jupiter (index) finger extended and the other fingers held down with the thumb. Grab the left Jupiter finger with the right hand making a fist around it.

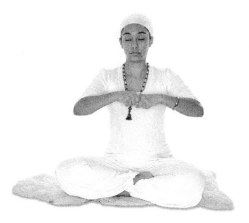

Holding this mudra, start moving the hands like a machine in small, tight forward circles in front of the Heart Center. Make about 6- to 9-inch circles. Move fast—at your maximum speed. Keep going—so fast that you get out of breath within 3 minutes. Get wild. You'll be totally exhausted when it finishes. The natural cosmos energy will replace the fatigue—which is the human bind.

TIME: 9 minutes.

TO END: Inhale deeply, suspend the breath and keep moving—this is the most positive moment. Hold the breath and move harder and faster. **15 seconds**. Keep moving and exhale completely. Inhale and really move. **10 seconds**. Keep moving and exhale. Inhale and hold. **10 seconds**. Exhale and move on to the next exercise.

(continued on next page)

PART THREE

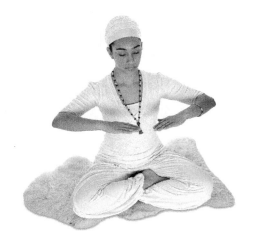

MUDRA & MOVEMENT: Without a rest, raise the elbows and arms to the level of the Heart Center. The elbows are bent with the forearms angled slightly. The thumb and fingers of each hand are together and the palms are flat and facing down. Keeping the angle of the arms, move from the shoulders so that the hands alternately cross over and under each other. Start with the left hand above the right. You have to move 120 times per minute—twice a second. Move fast and powerfully. You are creating the control of your magnetic field. Whatever magnetic field you create now is going to live with you as a permanent gain.

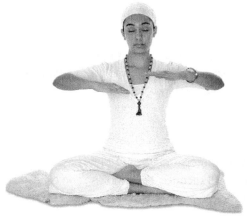

EYES: The eyes are closed. The concentration is very unique.

TIME: 4 minutes.

TO END: Inhale deeply and keep moving— harder and faster. Do your best. **15 seconds.** Exhale and inhale—keep moving. Don't stop. **15 seconds.** Exhale and inhale—keep moving. **10 seconds.** Exhale and inhale—still moving. **10 seconds.** Exhale and relax.

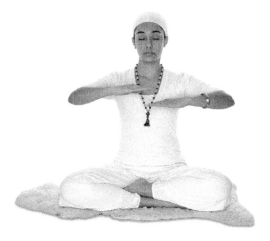

COMMENTS: The Jupiter energy in us is the energy that gives us civilization. It helps us understand our life. Jupiter is responsible for our prosperity, our purity and our powerful projection. You are dealing with a simple planet with a simple projection. Your complete focus makes a difference. Concentrate on your Jupiter finger and feel the phrase: "Proper power and prosperity."

Sometimes we need to make a conscious effort beyond our belief, beyond our knowledge and beyond our faith to check what we are doing to ourselves. We don't understand something that is actually very normal. First you have habits. Then the habits are you. If your habits are you, you no longer have your own identity. Know that your habits are not you. Your habits are an experienced way of living. They should not be automatic.

All the greatness is in your body, in your own self. You can't get it from outside. You have to create it from inside so that you can share with the outside and be popular and healthy and loving.

In the meditation, it's your own magnetic field that is causing all this pain and the work you are doing is healing you. It's a self-surgery. Go through the pain and don't stop.

This healing energy will be with you for a long time. Afterwards, you have to be very careful. That's why we seldom do this kind of exercise. When you create your own magnetic field, it can react to all other living beings' psyches. So be careful when you drive, be careful when you walk, be careful when you work, be careful when you open the door. Anything that moves while you move—be a little careful because you are very attractive now.

The original power of a person is not ordinary. Whenever we believe we are ordinary people, it's not true. We are very extra-ordinary. We all have a unique power, and it will stimulate in you your own uniqueness. It's not coming from outside. It triggers things that you have never understood or done before.

PURIFY THE SUBCONSCIOUS

January 14, 1989

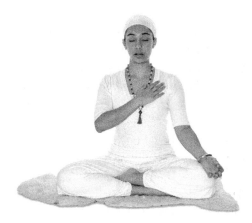

POSTURE: Sit in Easy Pose.

EYE FOCUS: The eyes are closed. Focus at the tip of the nose.

MUDRA: Using your intuition, choose a mudra for the left hand and place it at the knee. Place the right hand over the heart on the upper left chest.

MANTRA: Chant the mantra. Chant with the tongue, not the mouth.

Har Har Har Har Gobinday
Har Har Har Har Mukanday
Har Har Har Har Udaaray
Har Har Har Har Apaaray
Har Har Har Har Hareeang
Har Har Har Har Kareeang
Har Har Har Har Nirnaamay
Har Har Har Har Akaamay

TIME: 5 to 11 minutes.

GUIDELINES FOR PRACTICE: Practice the meditation for **5 to 11** minutes before going to bed. Then sleep with the mantra playing through the night. The following morning, before you get out of bed, chant this mantra. Sleep with this mantra and wake up with this mantra.

COMMENTS: In the tongue, the pair of *nadis* called the *ida* and *pingala* meet with the central *nadi*, the *shushmana*. That is the only place where the three powers meet—*ida*, *pingala* and *shushmana*; nowhere else is that union possible. Everywhere else they crisscross each other; the tongue is the only place where all three are straight. When you chant this mantra it will create an experience of unison—an intercourse, a merger—and you will be happy. So chant with your tongue not with your mouth.

It takes about 30 seconds to chant this. So, in one minute you can chant this whole *Ashtang Mantra* twice. There are eight powers described in these words—the eight facets of God that you have to deal with, whether you like it or not: *Gobinday*, one who sustains us; *Mukanday*, one who liberates us; Udaaray, one who takes us across, uplift us; *Apaaray*, one who is Infinite; *Hareeang*, one who does everything; *Kareeang*, one who by grace everything is done; *Nirnamay*, one who is not bound down, he is without the identity of the name; *Akaamay*, one who is by itself. These are the eight facets. HAR is a *Shakti Yog* mantra. HAR is the original God, and sometimes, if you chant just that one word, HAR, with me, you will realize God in just a couple of seconds.

When your subconscious hears this mantra at night, it will not allow for garbage. The subconscious will become pure. Acknowledge and practice this for **10-15 minutes** in the evening and in the morning; it will do the work. Learn one thing: become the hub and everything will come to you, become the rim and you will go everywhere. When you want two hundred thousand things, where are you going to go? You go crazy running this way and that way, and who cares? That's not living; that is hustling.

RECEIVING THE VIRTUES
July 25, 1989

PART ONE

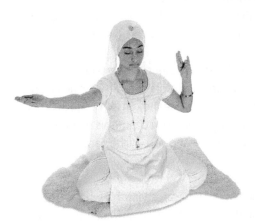

POSTURE: Sit straight in Easy Pose with a light Neck Lock.

EYE FOCUS: The eyes are closed. Concentrate behind the eyes—not at the Third Eye Point.

MUDRA: The left hand is by the shoulder (as if taking an oath), palm forward, with the thumb holding down the nail of the Sun Finger (ring finger). Keep the other fingers straight. Extend the right arm straight ahead and parallel to the ground, then raise the arm 15 degrees above parallel and move it to the right 60 degrees from the Heart Center (directly in front of you is 0 degrees; and directly to the right is 90 degrees). The palm is tilted up and the fingers are straight and together. Hold the mudra in silence. **3 minutes**.

Continue in the same posture listening to the music below. **14 minutes**.

MUSIC: *Bountiful, Blissful, Beautiful with Ek Ong Kaar Sat Gurprasad* by Nirinjan Kaur.

> *I am bountiful, blissful, and beautiful.*
> *Bountiful, blissful and beautiful I am.*
>
> *Ek ong kar sat gur prasad.*
> *Anand bhayaa*
> *mayree maa-ay*
> *Satguroo mai paa-yaa.*
> *Satigur ta paa-yaa*
> *sehej saytee*
> *Man vajeeaa vaadhaaeeaa.*
> *Raag ratan parvaar pareeaa shabad gaavan aaeeaa*
> *Shabado taa gaavho haree kayraa man jinee vasaa-yaa.*
> *Kahai naanak anand hoaa satiguroo mai paa-yaa.*

TRANSLATION:
The Creator and the Creation are One. I know this by the Grace of the Guru.
Oh my mother, I am in Infinite bliss for I have obtained the True Guru (the Word, the *Shabad Guru*)

I have met that True Guru easily, naturally Divine music bursts in my heart.
The rhythmic beats are like cosmic jewels and bring all powers through Divine Songs.
When God resides in you, the mind is filled by and echoes with divine praise.
Naanak proclaims I dwell in supreme bliss for I have merged with the True Guru.

TO END: Inhale deeply, suspend the breath and concentrate on the back of the eyes.
15 -30 seconds. Exhale. Repeat 3 times. Very slowly relax your hands down, palms facing up and begin Long Deep Breathing. **2 ½ Minutes.** Extend both hands up, arms straight up, and stretch. Shake the hands, move the spine. **30 seconds.**

COMMENTS: Let heaven drop virtues into the palm of your hand. From the closed eyes, concentrate behind your eyes—not at the third eye point—and feel the virtues dropping into your hands. The moment your virtues start coming, your hands will feel the gravity of lead, then the weight of silver, then gold, and finally platinum.

Part Two

MUDRA: Mercury (pinkie) finger and thumb together; thumb covers the nail of the Mercury finger in each hand. The arms are in the same position as Part One. **11 minutes.**

MUSIC: Chant with the musical version of *Ardas Bhaee* by Nirinjan Kaur.

TRANSLATION:

The prayer has been given to Guru Amar Das.

The prayer is manifested by Guru Ram Das.

The miracle is complete.

Ardaas Bhaee,
Amar Das Guroo
Amar Das Guru, Ardaas Bhaee
Raam Daas Guroo, Raam Daas Guroo
Raam Daas Guroo, Sachee Sahee

TO END: Inhale deeply, suspend the breath and repeat the mantra mentally **20 seconds**. Exhale. Repeat 3 times.

COMMENTS: When you lock the pinkie, you lock the earth. With both hands locked in this way, your meditation becomes an irrevocable prayer.

OUR PATTERN, PERSONALITY AND PROJECTION

September 10, 1995

PART ONE

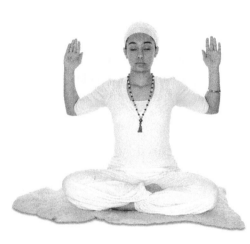

POSTURE: Come into Easy Pose. (Note: this set was taught to people sitting straight in their chairs, both feet equally weighted on the ground.)

MUDRA: Bend the forearms up so that the hands are facing forward with the fingers pointing upward. The elbows are elevated a little bit so that the hands are just outside of the shoulder area and must be positioned slightly behind the line of the earlobes for the full effect. The shoulder muscles must be pulled a little backwards and toward one another. If it starts hurting that means you are doing it right.

BREATH: One-minute breath. Concentrate on your breath and control it mechanically and silently. Inhale **20 seconds**. Suspend the breath **20 seconds**. Exhale **20 seconds**.

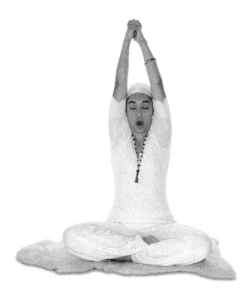

MANTRA: Listen to the mantra Sat Nam Wahe Guru, Indian Version #2, pronounced *SAT(I) NAAM, SAT(I) NAAM, WHAA-HAY GUROO WHAA-HAY GUROO* to provide a rhythm for the breath. But keep breathing in absolute silence.

TIME: 11 minutes.

END: Inhale deeply and suspend the breath. Raise the hands up over the head and interlock the fingers. Stretch the spine as much as you can **5 seconds**. Cannon fire out through the mouth. Repeat 2 more times. Relax.

COMMENTS: Whosoever perfects this breathing science with this posture can conquer one's own death.

Sit in absolute silence and don't worry. The hammer bone of your inner ear will bring changes. You don't have to do a thing. Just set yourself in perfect posture and breathe consciously. The rest will be taken care of.

Try not to hear the sound. Try to block the sound. Use your mental control to concentrate only on the breath and the posture.

PART TWO

POSTURE: Continue to sit peacefully in Easy Pose.

MUDRA: Make the hands into fists with the Jupiter (index) fingers extended and the thumbs holding down the other fingers.

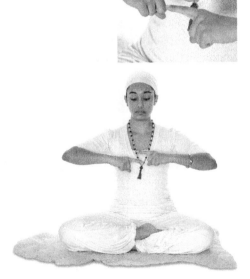

Bring the fists to the level of the Heart Center and face the two Jupiter fingers towards each other so that they are overlapping. Then begin to spin the fingers around each other without touching. They move fast—as fast as **3 times per second**, 180 times per minute.

EYE FOCUS: The eyes are open, looking down at the fingers.

TIME: 8 minutes.

COMMENTS: This second exercise will change the metabolism and the blood stream. The glandular system will secrete differently. We practice these exercises as a science—not as a mythology. To us, there is no mystery. It's a well-known, organized, scientific reality. Every person has the right to progress and every progressive self has to have a definite discipline, to create a frequency and a projection. To us, that is God.

(continued on next page)

This is a very funny exercise. You will laugh at it, but do it fully and you will understand why you are doing it. The Jupiter finger is a finger of wisdom and tranquility. It is your power to overpower your negativity or somebody else's negativity. Bear the pain. This is Jupiter. The western and eastern hemispheres of the brain will start correlating at the neutral place so you don't want the fingers to touch. That's how it is. The exercise will change your breathing. It will change your thinking. And it will change your mental projection. Because it will recharge your brain energy and bring equilibrium to both hemispheres of the brain, left and right. But you have to look at the fingers and you have to go fast.

After a couple of minutes you are going to go crazy—that's what it does. You must build stamina to keep up. Your ego cannot tolerate that you cannot do this little exercise. This is where you win.

You couldn't do in eleven years what this exercise can do in eleven minutes. You can do eleven minutes of this exercise. Another person can go and sit on a rock for eleven years. The man who sits on the rock will be as dumb as he started and you will be fine, because the power is inside us. We have to work with our neurological system.

PART THREE

Keeping up in the posture, begin to whistle and slow down the movement of the fingers. Move the Jupiter fingers slowly. Whistle and move your fingers to the rhythm of your own whistle. In this third part we deeply meditate and touch our inner self, our soul.

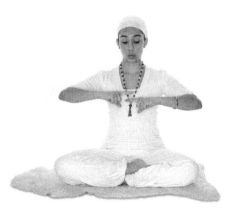

TIME: 3 minutes.

Inhale deeply. Bring your hands into prayer pose at the Heart Center. Inhale through the nose and exhale through the mouth very strongly. Clear out all sickness and disease, and your inferiority complex. Become your own healer. 1 ½ minutes.

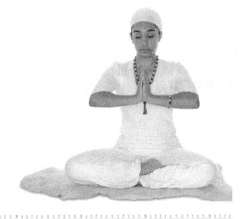

TO END: Inhale deeply and press your hands against each other with maximum pressure. **10 seconds**. Exhale. Inhale again, and again press. **5 seconds**. Exhale. Inhale a third time applying maximum pressure with the hands. **5 seconds**. Exhale.

COMMENTS: There is a part in the hemispheres of our brain called the third neurological plate cycle that sets the pattern of our personality. In one hundred years, medically, they are going to figure this out. There is a little stem of the brain—they don't know what it does. But it has three rings to set your temperament, your metabolism and your pattern.

This meditation works on the third neurological plate that sets our pattern, our personality and our projection. The exercise is not very beautiful because it will move you and it will shake you up. It is not fashionable; it requires you to work. But, God, if you can take that dead part of you out, you will be living again.

The effectiveness of your personality shows in how you speak. When you wake up in the morning and you open your eyes to be yourself, that first minute sets the whole frequency of the day. If you get up one day feeling indifferent toward yourself for that first minute, everything you encounter will be indifferent to you the whole day. There is nothing wrong with you, but the frequency of your psyche and the frequency of the psyche of the day will not connect.

These exercises are very simple. Through them, we work with certain muscles and meridian points. We stimulate the reaction in the hemisphere of the brain and we cause fear. And then we ask the master part of the brain, through the medulla, to coordinate and correct the fear. Thus, we develop the automatic system of corrective behavior within ourselves.

When you do these exercises, they are very simple. They are very simple but after a while they will become very painful. The normal tendency at that time is not to do it. At that moment you have to win. After a while you will come out of the pain and you will be in a different space. If you continue doing these three exercises every day, you can set the pace of your personality to invoke in you the self-power.

If you can do these three exercises in your lifetime, you will never be hurt. It only takes forty days to perfect yourself. This exercise will not give you a chance for foolish thinking. If you do this exercise, after forty days, you will never space out. It doesn't matter what happens—even under hypnosis you will not space out. We used to give this exercise to our intelligence staff so if they got caught and put under hypnosis, they would have self-control.

THE PROSPERITY MANTRA
April 15, 2000

Har Har Har Har
Gobinday
Har Har Har Har
Mukhanday
Har Har Har Har Har
Udaaray
Har Har Har Har
Apaaray
Har Har Har Har
Hareeang
Har Har Har Har
Kareeang
Har Har Har Har
Nirnaamay
Har Har Har Har
Akaamay

This mantra fixes the mind to prosperity and power. It contains the eight facets of the Self with Har, the original force of Creativity. The four repetitions of Har give power to all aspects and provide the power to break down the barriers of the past. It converts fear into the determination to use and expand the reserve energy of the Navel Point. It invokes guidance and sustenance; all powers come to serve your true purpose.

"The four *HARS* are combined with the *Guru Gaitri Mantra*. *GOBINDAY*—Sustaining; *MUKANDAY*—Liberating; *UDAARAY*—Enlightening; *APAARAY*—Infinite; *HAREEANG*— Destroying; *KAREEANG*—Creating; *NIRNAAMAY*—Nameless; *AKAAMAY*—Desireless.[48]
Yogi Bhajan translated the Guru Gaitri Mantra as follows:

One who sustains us.
One who liberates us.
One who uplifts us.
Infinite One.
One who does everything.
One by whose grace everything is done.
Nameless and desireless.
Encompasses all.

48 Adapted from *The Aquarian Teacher*.

MUDRAS TO USE WITH THE PROSPERITY MANTRA:

When it is chanted on the communication line of Mercury (Buddhi Mudra—the tips of the pinkie fingers and thumbs touch), it is for friendship and prosperity. When chanted on sun line (Surya Mudra—the tips of the ring fingers and thumbs touch), it is for health. When it is chanted on the Saturn line (Shuni Mudra—the tips of the middle fingers and thumbs touch), it is for purity and piety. When it is chanted on the Jupiter line (Gyan Mudra—the tips of the forefingers and thumbs touch), then hurdles disappear.

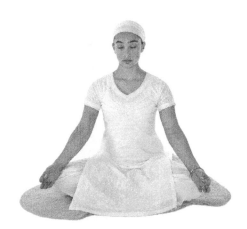

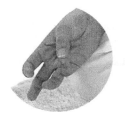 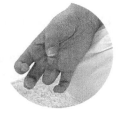 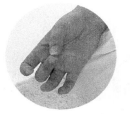 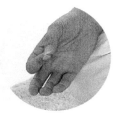

This mantra has a forty-sound resound system in it. It affects the seven chakras and the eighth, the arc line of the human (also known as the aura) in the five *tattvas* of ether, air, water, earth and fire. It has the strength of forty, such that it can penetrate through any negativity, any misfortune. It has the power to break through—no matter what. We have seen it. It has come through for centuries. There is nothing new about it. It is not very secret but it is very, very sacred.

MEDITATION FOR MENTAL CLARITY AND PURITY

Published in *Prosperity Paths* in December, 1998

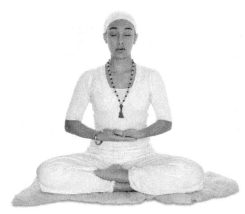

POSTURE: Sit in Easy Pose or in a chair with the weight of both feet equally distributed on the ground.

MUDRA: For men, rest the right hand in the left with both hands facing up. For women, the position is reversed. Point both thumbs straight away from the body. Hold this position at the center of the chest, at the curve of the rib cage. The arms rest against the sides of the body with the elbows bent.

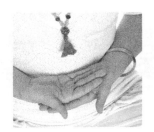

EYES: The eyes are almost completely closed.

MANTRA: In the above position, begin chanting the mantra.

GOBIND GOBIND, HAREE HAREE

Continue the chant without any breaks, allowing the breath to regulate itself.

Chant the mantra in a monotone, in a four-beat rhythm. As you say, "Go" pucker your lips as if to kiss someone, and relax them on the syllable "Bind."

TIME: No restrictions were placed on the length of time this can be practiced.

COMMENTS: This meditation has the capacity to make your mind clear as crystal. It can totally eliminate mental impurity, but it must be done correctly. In the coming times, many people will become nervous wrecks. They will not even be in a position to receive instruction in meditation. All you will be able to do for them is to put your hands over their heads and start chanting. This meditation will help to develop the healing powers within you, provided you also perfect the mantra *SAA TAA NAA MAA RAA MAA DAA SAA SAA SAY SO HANG*.

MAHAN KAAL KRIYA

April 30, 1973

"This kriya will bring innocence and dispel fear from the personality. It is very powerful. If it is practiced, everyone in your family will live to a ripe old age." —Yogi Bhajan

POSTURE: Sit in Easy Pose.

MUDRA: Cross your hands on your chest and pull *Maha Bhand* (tuck the chin back, pull up and in on the anus, sex organs, Navel Point and diaphragm). Look back and up to the top of the head. Pain will come to the side of the jaws.

MANTRA: In the center of the head, vibrate the mantra.

AKAAL

MAHAA

KAAL

TRANSLATION:
Timelessness,
Great Expansive
Time.

TIME: Unlimited.

COMMENTS: It is my study that all divorces are caused by one thing only—clash of ego. And every clash of ego has arisen out of fear. Have faith. Only one thing is the enemy—our past experiences. These lead to guilt complexes that are recorded in our subconscious mind and then we relate with complexes according to our past. We believe in saving face, not the soul.

Man suffers for one reason: he loses his innocence. When you lose your innocence, you end up with disputes. The idea of this yoga is to regain innocence so that universal consciousness will serve you and maintain you. When your doubts are gone, then your fears will be gone and your feelings and experiences will be of happiness.

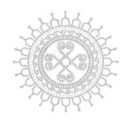

Refining the Mind and Developing Intuition

INTUITION

April 24, 1991

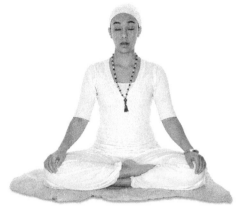

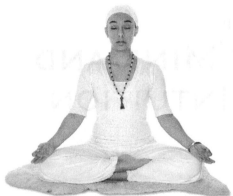

POSTURE: Sit as a yogi—as your exalted self.

EYES: The eyes are closed.

MENTAL FOCUS: Concentrate between the eyebrows and the root of the nose. Just concentrate deeper and deeper until you reach self-hypnosis—the point where everything of you is gone. Only the pituitary point and you live. Concentrate. Amalgamate yourself. Accelerate your hypnotic trance created by the Self. Go deeper and deeper and deeper.

MUSIC & MANTRA: The gong is played. Simultaneously, *Ang Sang Wahe Guru*—the musical affirmation by Nirinjan Kaur—is played. The musical affirmation is just loud enough that it can be heard when the gong sound starts to fade.

ANG SANG WHAA-HAY GUROO

TRANSLATION: The dynamic, loving energy of the Infinite Source of All is dancing within my every cell, and is present in my every limb. My individual consciousness merges with the Universal consciousness.

The combined gong and *Ang Sang Wahe Guru* is played for **9 minutes.** Then the gong stops, but the musical affirmation continues.

Slowly and gradually return to the sound of the mantra. Listen to *Ang Sang Wahe Guru*, then whisper it, then chant it.

TIMING: Close the eyes and concentrate—get into a self-hypnotic state in silence, **3 minutes**.
Gong is played with *Ang Sang Wahe Guru*, **9 minutes**.
Gong ends. Continue listening. **1 ½ minutes**.
Whisper, **6 minutes**.
Chant out loud, **2 ½ minutes**.
Total time for meditation is **22 minutes**.

TO END: Inhale deeply and tighten the whole body. Take the tongue and press the upper palate. Press it hard. **15 seconds**. Let it go. Inhale again, deeply. Press the upper palate hard. **15 seconds**. Let it go. Inhale deeply. Press the tongue against the upper palate. Harder, harder, harder. **30 seconds**. Relax.

COMMENTS: We will play a one-half, a two-and-three-quarter, and a three-and-a-half cycle rhythm to penetrate through the sound. In the hypnotic sense, this sound can give you an experience of Infinity that you cannot otherwise measure.

It is the impotency of karma that takes you away from *dharma*. You start the sequence of consequences and finally you lose the game. Why? Because you do not have your intuition under your control. The divine guidance is not there. Whenever a man is guided by his ego, insult in the court of God is guaranteed. "*Dharam na vidah, homeh nal varodh heh*. God's kingdom has a direct animosity with ego." Ego and divinity will never walk together. Where you burn a candle darkness will go away, but put out the candle and darkness will come back. Why do we need intuition? We need it every moment. Why? Because we want to know. If we don't know, we have to hustle. And all our precious life is wasted in hustling.

Are you even enough to survive against every odd? There is only one way to do it. You must have your own intuition, and your spirit must talk to you.

This recording tonight is my gift to you. We'll name it "Intuition." The word intuition has a preface. It will cut across human rationality and logic, and set you on faith. If you practice it for 40 days, you will start seeing the results.

It is my dedication to the renaissance that started America on the road to being America again[49]. It is my reverence to twenty million young Americans who started with the call of the soul and who sacrificed their lives so that, in this country, mankind would live from maya to dharma. It is my dedication to those who survived with their commitment and keep the banner today. May it live to continue to the last breath of their lives.

---

49 Yogi Bhajan is referring to the Cultural Revolution of the 60s.

SHIV KARNI KRIYA
WITH IK ACHAREE CHAND SHABAD

April 30, 2001

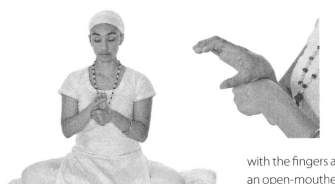

POSTURE: Sit straight in Easy Pose.

MUDRA: Make a tight fist of the left hand and rest the wrist of the right hand on top of it, facing forward, with the fingers and thumb tightly arched like an open-mouthed snake ready to strike. Place this mudra in front of the Heart Center. Elbows are relaxed down.

EYE FOCUS: Eyes are 1/10th open and focused at the tip of the nose.

MANTRA: Chant the *Ik Acharee Chand shabad* using the recording by Gurushabad Singh and Nirinjan Kaur

Ajai Alai	Invincible, Indestructible
Abhai Abai	Fearless, Unchanging
Abhoo Ajoo	Unformed, Unborn
Anaas Akaas	Imperishable, Etheric
Aganj Abhanj	Unbreakable, Impenetrable
Alakh Abhakh	Unseen, Unaffected
Akaal Dyaal	Undying, Merciful
Alaykh Abhaykh	Indescribable, Uncostumed
Anaam Akaam	Nameless, Desireless
Agaahaa Adhaahaa	Unfathomable, Incorruptible
Anaathay Pramaathay	Unmastered, Destroyer
Ajonee Amonee	Beyond birth, Beyond silence
Na Raagay Na Rangay	Beyond love, Beyond color
Na Roopay Na Raykhay	Beyond form, Beyond shape
Akaramang Abharamang	Beyond karma, Beyond doubt
Aganjay Alaykhay	Unconquerable, Indescribable

TIME: 31 minutes.

TO END: Inhale and hold briefly. Exhale and relax.

COMMENTS: Understand Guru Nanak's words, *Ek Ong Kaar*, "The universe is created by the One, and you are part of that One." Have patience and wait. Things will start happening. All prosperity is based on opportunity, though you believe opportunity has to be caught. But it will only happen when the Hand of the Creator is behind it, not when you involve your ego.

The ultimate knowledge of the Age of Aquarius is that *purkha* is the source of *prakriti*.

Chanting *Ajai Alai* with this mudra is like releasing an arrow from a bowstring. Without this mudra it is like throwing an arrow with the hand. This mudra makes a heavenly difference.

FOR WEALTH AND INTUITIVE OPPORTUNITY

February 2, 1976

PART ONE: WARM UPS

POSTURE: Sit in Easy Pose.

MUDRA: Relax your arms at your sides with your palms facing forward. Alternately bend each elbow, bringing the palms toward the center of your chest, but do not touch your chest. Do not bend the wrists or hands. Move as rapidly as you can and maintain a balance in the rhythmic motion of your hands. **3-11 minutes**.

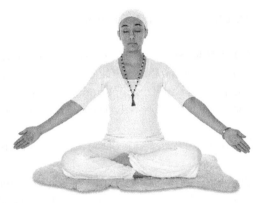

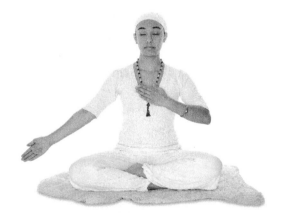

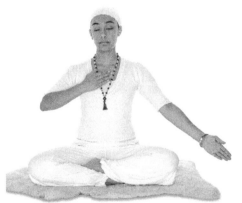

PART TWO: MEDITATION

POSTURE: Sit in Easy Pose.

MUDRA: Lightly connect the fingertips of the left and right hands to equalize the energy, leaving the thumbs separated and extended toward the Heart Center. The fingers are loosely separated and the hands are relaxed. The thumbs must not touch.

EYE FOCUS: Look down through your hands at a 60-degree angle.

MANTRA: Chant *Hareeang* **16 times** per breath. The chanting cycle takes about 13-15 seconds. **11-31 minutes**.

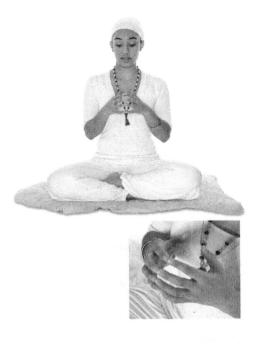

COMMENTS: It may take a couple of months to bring this meditation under your control, but if you do this meditation for 90 days, it can activate your brain so that you can know exactly what is what. It can make it intuitively possible for you to live creatively to your own potential and to tap the opportunities around you.

TRIGGER THE POSITIVE MIND
January 10, 1998

"If you are really positive about it, then the positive mind may serve you forever."

— Yogi Bhajan

PART ONE

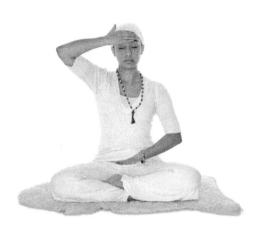

POSTURE: In Easy Pose, take your left hand, put it under your shirt and find your Navel Point and place the center of your palm over it. Take your right hand and put your four fingers on the forehead, thumb sticking up.

BREATH: Breathe mechanically, not automatically. Breathe yourself. Breathe in yourself. Breathe in mechanically, breathe out mechanically. Keep your spine straight, keep your contact points on the forehead and Navel Center and see what happens.

TIME: 7 minutes.

COMMENTS: Between your Navel Point and your Agia Chakra, or *ajna*—the Third Eye. I am not saying what will happen. It's a simple, scientific challenge. Your head is up there. Your heart is in-between. And your Navel Point is the basic nucleus of what the Chinese call your chi energy. We call it your ji energy, your "I" energy, or the center *shushmana* from where, as a spermatazoa and egg, you took this body, this shape and your geography. You grew, you lived and you enjoyed without taking a breath of life. You were born and this Navel Point provided you everything—remember that. So this energy is the immortal energy, not the mortal energy.

In yoga, never breathe the breath of life automatically. Always breathe mechanically. 31 minutes of mechanical breathing can give you health like you have never had. It can give you strength like you have never understood. It can give you answers for every question—even questions you cannot fathom. Because you live by the breath; you die by the breath. So you must enjoy the breath.

Part Two

POSTURE: Take your left hand and put it around the back of your neck, holding the neck in this grip. Place the right hand at the Heart Center.

EYES: The eyes are closed.

BREATH: Inhale mechanically through whichever nostril is working and exhale through the mouth.

TIME: 10 minutes

COMMENTS: You have all the Cs, 1-6, under your hand (vertebra in the neck). That neck grip means that the blood will rush, the spinal serum will rush, and your brain will get an automatic tonic. Press your heart. Press it to the point where you can feel the vibrations at the forehead. Check it out.

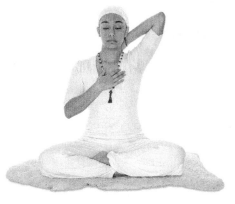

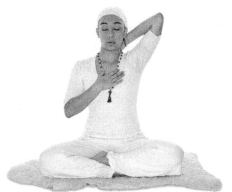

(continued on next page)

PART THREE

POSTURE: Stay in the position and begin to whistle to *Ardas Bhaee*[50]. You will find the rhythm and it will automatically elevate you. Project the energy as you contain your biorhythmic psyche.

TIME: 3 minutes.

TO END: Relax.

COMMENTS: The work is that your mind has to be positive. The positive mind has to tell you, "I am made in the likeness of God or the Creator," (if you are atheist, say anything, it doesn't matter)." I am made in something and I have to prove to something, I am beautiful, bountiful, I am in bliss." You can only live absolutely happily if you build a positive mind.

The only way you can become independent is if you are intuitive. And to develop your intuition, you have to have your breath—the basic elementary power of life—under your control. And you must have a positive mind because all the thoughts that are stuck in the subconscious will start dropping into the unconscious when it's overloaded—and then you will have nightmares. So you have to get rid of them at the subconscious level.

You must achieve things through the mind—the positive mind. Achieve positive things for yourself. When you are positive, your life is positive, your projection is positive. Then you will find a lot of people love you, a lot of people come to you. There are two ways to live, folks. One is to hustle and live. The other is to live and let things come to you. So if your magnetic psyche can be positively aroused from point six, point eight, point nine or one to two point five, everything in the world you ever need mentally, subconsciously, consciously or unconsciously will come to you. If you really are positive about it, then the positive mind may serve you forever.

---

[50] Recordings of **Ardas Bhaee** can be purchased from Ancient Healing Ways or Spirit Voyage.

One-Minute Breath[51]

Come into a meditative posture. Inhale for **20 seconds**. Hold for **20 seconds.** Exhale for **20 seconds**.

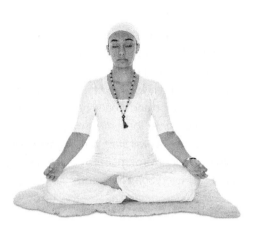

Physiological effects of the one-minute breath include: optimized cooperation between the brain hemispheres, dramatic calming of anxiety, fear and worry, openness to feeling one's presence and the presence of spirit, stronger intuition, whole-brain functioning—especially the old brain and the frontal hemispheres. –Yogi Bhajan, from *The Aquarian Teacher*

"On average, you breathe twenty to twenty-five breaths per minute. In good health you breathe ten times a minute and a mentally balanced person breathes seven to nine breaths per minute. Fewer than that and you are a yogi.

"If you want things to be done for you so you don't have to do anything, then you must breathe from one to five or six breaths per minute. If you can practice that, then you can attract the universe to you. It is no secret. It's a simple thing. The longer and deeper your breath is, the more your psyche attracts everything to you—it's a way to prosperity.

"If you sit down and breathe one breath a minute, in exactly thirty seconds you will find you are talking to yourself. In three minutes, you can get over any kind of mood. Why are you suffering? Do you want to live a long time? If you breathe an average of fifteen times a minute, and you live one hundred years. If instead you breathe one breath a minute, you can live fifteen hundred years because life is measured by the breath, not by years or by the calendar. When you are unconscious, your breath will be shallow and strong. But if you practice one breath a minute for eleven minutes a day, you can be in your control of your mind.

"Twenty seconds to inhale, twenty seconds to hold, twenty seconds to let it out. It takes one minute. And if you just practice from eleven minutes to thirty-one minutes, your blood itself will become a warrior against disease.

(continued on next page)

---

[51]   These comments were taken from lectures given by Yogi Bhajan on September 10, 1995 and November 10, 2001.

"I told one person, 'For thirty-one minutes do the one-minute breath meditation.' It's the story of man who is grateful today; who is successful today; who has become compassionate without any lecture. He has realized himself. Why? It's so simple. You live by breath, you die by breath. And if you meditate on your breath, the *Pavan Guru*, the knowledge of the *pranic vidya* of creation and creativity and all incarnations will dawn on you. For some people it may take a short time, for some it may take a long time. But the path is the same. The procedure is the same. You will start winning yourself. You will start valuing your breath. You will start valuing your environments. You will start valuing your projections and one day you will be surprised. Everyone will, in turn, value you."

I, MY MIND, WE, THOU, THEE

June 19, 1998

MUDRA: Bring the forearms parallel to the ground in front of the Heart Center, palms facing down. Place the right hand over the left, lightly touching. The fingertips of the right hand are at the edge of the left wrist. The fingertips of the left hand touch the underside of the right wrist.

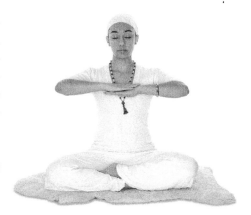

MANTRA: Chant the mantra in a monotone from the navel.

I
MY MIND
WE
THOU
THEE

Yogi Bhajan demonstrated the mantra in a specific 8-beat rhythm giving each word a solid beat with 2 silent beats as follows:

I—my—mind—(beat)—we—thou—thee—(beat)

TIME: 9 ½ minutes.

TO END: Inhale deeply, suspend the breath **15 seconds** and listen to what you have said. Let the mantra be your only thought. Exhale. Inhale again. Suspend the breath and hold the thought **15 seconds**. Exhale. Inhale again and allow the sounds of those words to come to your ears. Suspend the breath **15 seconds** and exhale and relax.

COMMENTS: Practice this meditation so you can walk the distance, reach your destiny and make many to follow you.

You do not know the basic formula of life. I, My Mind, We, Thou, Thee. That is what *Anand Sahib*[52] is all about. It's the Guru's given wisdom between a man and his mind, a man and his body, and a man and his spirit. Anybody can adopt it. Anybody can understand it. Anybody can work with it and live in bliss.

---

[52] *Anand Sahib* is the *Song of Bliss*—a sacred teaching written by the third Sikh Master, Guru Amar Das, who lived in the 16th century.

MEDITATION TO DELIVER CONTENTMENT

PART ONE

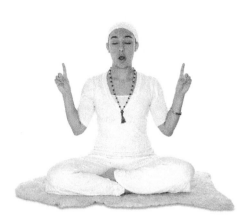

POSTURE: Sit straight in Easy Pose.

MUDRA: Raise both hands to shoulder level, palms facing forward, with the elbows relaxed down. Point the index fingers up and hold the other fingers with the thumbs.

EYES: The eyes are closed.

BREATH: Conscious, slow, Long Deep Breathing through the "O" of your mouth.

TIME: 11 minutes.

PART TWO

Continue with the same posture and deepen the breath even more, pulling the navel toward the spine with each exhale. Meditate on your mind. Achieve a state where your mind remains balanced despite what anybody says. If you count your values, you give your virtues a chance, and vice-versa.

TIME: 11 minutes.

TO END: Inhale deeply, hold and squeeze your spine, muscle by muscle. Exhale. Repeat 2 times, on the last breath squeezing every part of your body from head to toe. Relax.

COMMENTS BY DR. GURUCHANDER SINGH KHALSA:

For each of us on the path, there are two qualities that must be present if we are to achieve a life of prosperity—a life that is pro-spirit. The first quality is containment, which creates an opportunity to deliver oneself to the second quality—a state of contentment.

This meditation can deliver both aspects: containment and contentment. It creates a direct connection to the radiant body—our largest aura—and gives us control of the mind. Control of our mind gives us the opportunity to allow contentment as a choice, a state of being to be assimilated into our daily awareness as a dominant feature of our psyche.

ATTITUDE OF GRATITUDE
June 26, 1998

POSTURE: Sit in Easy Pose with a straight spine, chin in, chest out, belly in. Physically and mentally straighten your spine, so the channels can be clear.

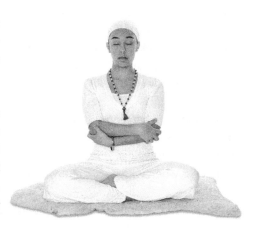

MUDRA: Bend the elbows down by the sides and cross the forearms over the diaphragm area, parallel to the floor, right on top, left underneath. Grab the right elbow with the left hand and the left elbow with the right hand. Comfortably lock your hands so that you have the elbows in your hands.

EYES: The eyes are closed.

BREATH: Breathe long and deep for **1 to 2 minutes** before beginning to chant.

MANTRA:

Har Har Har Har Gobinday
Har Har Har Har Mukanday
Har Har Har Har Udaaray
Har Har Har Har Apaaray
Har Har Har Har Hareeang
Har Har Har Har Kareeang
Har Har Har Har Nirnaamay
Har Har Har Har Akaamay

Nirinjan Kaur's version was used in class. See translation on page 184.

Chant the mantra out loud from the navel. **1 minute.**
Whisper powerfully. Use the *pranic* power. Keep the navel engaged. **3 ½ minutes**.
Then chant silently. Move the breath with the navel. Keep the navel moving as if you were chanting—but you are silently chanting with the mantra. **8 minutes.**

TO END: Inhale deeply, stretch your spine as much as you can, while squeezing the ribcage, the area where your elbows are locked, as well as every part of your body. Hold **15-20 seconds**. Cannon Fire exhale through the mouth. Repeat for a total of **3 times**. Relax.

(continued on next page)

COMMENTS: All this knowledge is ancient and it is forgotten. We who practice Kundalini Yoga have no right to initiate anyone. Because if somebody cannot initiate himself or herself, we should not be so foolish as to initiate that person. Basically, the law is that you have to be you to start with. And then you grow. Because you have three parts: a demon part, a human part and an angelic part. At the very least you should accept yourself—you are human. Don't talk negative, think negative, let anybody down, or participate in any let down. You should always be aware that any negative word you say negates you a hundred times more than it negates anybody else.

What happens when you speak positively? When you speak positively there is no negative left to express and then there's a gap. And that gap creates the super-positive. And that, in English, is what we call God. Therefore, cultivate the attitude of gratitude. The attitude of gratitude is when you are grateful for every breath of life.

People ask me, "What should we do when we feel something is wrong?" When there is something wrong, thank God it is not you. When you feel there is something good, thank God that you have learned something. In this way, you can process your life and progress your life.

What will happen? You will get high-spirited. You will rise. And, to fill the vacuum, nature will come with wealth and prosperity. Otherwise your poverty is proportionate to your emotionalism and your bad relationships and bad sex and bad marriage are equal to your commotionalism. These are forces. I am not saying get rid of them, I am saying they will get rid of you. There is nothing you can do.

Some people are the most inhuman idiots. They are so insecure about everything. They have not learned that God—who can rotate this earth for you, creating day and night—can take care of your routine if you allow it to be. But you don't allow it.

We do not want to know how good we are. We want to know how bad everybody else is, but we can never, ever find our goodness this way. If somebody is bad, let it be. But try not to be bad yourself.

We have a very good mantra that creates prosperity. Mantra is *"man" "tra."* It is a mentally projected vibration that entangles with Infinity and creates the effect. It is a sound system that you, I, me, we, they, thou can all create. It has nothing to do with what you feel or what you are. But when all the vibrations of you and your environments have gone negative, that is the moment to use the mantra. When you chant this mantra with the breath of life, you tap into all the angels of the Universe, including your own great ancestors who have a qualifying life as an angel. It's quick. It's fast. It's purposeful. It brings in what you need.

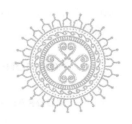

PART FOUR

THE POWER OF THE WORD

ACTIVATE THE POWER OF COMMUNICATION

August 22, 1986

"Learn to be alert. Answer with the power of the soul. Relate with an affirmation. Every word you say should be an affirmation." —Yogi Bhajan

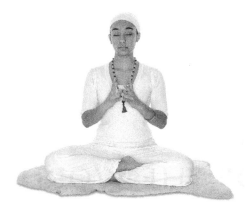

POSITION: Sit in Easy Pose.

MUDRA: Touch the thumb and Mercury (pinkie) finger of one hand to the thumb and Mercury finger of the other hand. Bend the Sun (ring) fingers in toward the palms, but do not let them touch the palms. Leave the Jupiter (index) and Saturn (middle) fingers pointing straight up, but not touching. Place the mudra 3 to 4 inches in front of the Heart Center.

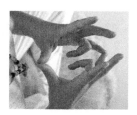

TIME: Start with **11 minutes** and work up to **31 minutes**.

MANTRA: Meditatively listen to *Beloved God*[53], the first song on Singh Kaur's Peace Lagoon recording.

*Beloved God,
May the precious flowers
of my devotion
Blossom in the gardens
of Thy heart.
While I await the dawn
of Thy coming.*

[53] This is a translation of a stanza from *Sukhmani Sahib* in the English *Peace Lagoon*.

EXCEL, EXCEL, FEARLESS

POSTURE: Sit in Easy Pose, with a straight spine.

MUDRA: Hands are in Gyan Mudra (tips of the index finger and the thumb touching each other, forming a circle), wrists on the knees.

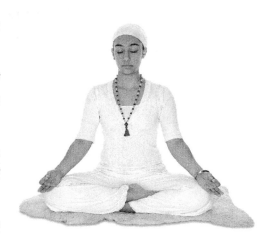

EYES: Look at the center of your chin, through closed eyes. Or focus at the tip of your nose with your eyes 1/10th open.

MANTRA: Inhale deeply, suspend the breath and mentally recite:

I AM BOUNTIFUL.
I AM BLISSFUL.
I AM BEAUTIFUL.

Exhale completely and hold the breath out as you mentally recite:

EXCEL, EXCEL, FEARLESS.

TIME: Practice **3 minutes** at a time a couple of times a day.

25TH PAURI OF JAPJI SAHIB (BAHUTA KARAM)

"If you recite the 25th *Pauri* of *Japji* 11 times a day, it will bring you prosperity and wealth."
— Yogi Bhajan

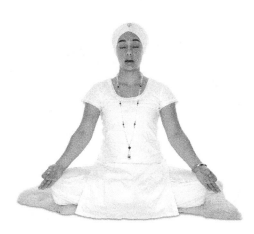

POSTURE: Sit in Easy Pose, with a straight spine.

MUDRA: The hands are resting on the knees in Gyan Mudra (first fingers and thumb tips are touching).

EYES: The eyes may be open or closed.

MANTRA: The 25th *Pauri* of *Japji Sahib*. (See page 212)

TIME: 11 times.

COMMENTS: If you recite the 25th *pauri* of *Japji* 11 times a day, it will bring you prosperity and wealth. It is a promise. There are many people who have done it and they became prosperous.

The 25th *pauri* adds up to seven. It is a platform of levitation. It means wherever you are and whatever you are, this *pauri* will elevate you, levitate you, to the point of achievement, no matter what!

Prosperity is a state produced immediately by the mind. When the sun comes out of the clouds, everything is lit. When the mind comes out of duality, prosperity is there. And the 25th *pauri* has the power to take away duality, because it covers every aspect of the projection of the self. It works on the tenth body, the Radiant Body.

25ᵀᴴ PAURI OF JAPJI SAHIB WITH MUDRA

April 23, 1997

"This *shabad* will change poverty to prosperity." — Yogi Bhajan

PART ONE

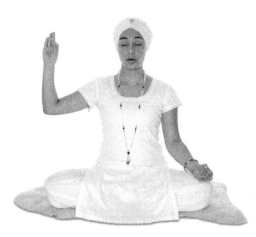

POSITION: Sit in Easy Pose with a straight spine.

MUDRA: Bring both hands into Gyan Mudra (touch the tip of the index finger with the tip of the thumb, the other fingers remain straight). Place the right hand, palm facing forward, next to the shoulder. The fingers point up with the hand at the level of the face. The left elbow is bent and the left hand rests on the left knee, palm facing up.

EYES: The eyes are closed.

MANTRA: Chant the *25th Pauri of Japji Sahib* aloud. (See page 212) **31 minutes.**

PART TWO

Remain in the same posture. Breathe very long, deep and slow through the nose. In the silence, hear the sound of the mantra in your inner ear. **5 minutes.**

TO END: Inhale deeply and squeeze your entire spine from top to bottom, bringing the energy from the Earth to the Heavens. Hold for **15-20 seconds.** Cannon fire exhale through the mouth. Repeat **2 more times.** Relax.

NOTE: It is recommended to dance for a few minutes after completing this meditation to balance out the energy and keep the nervous system strong. Yogi Bhajan played bhangara music for this purpose.

25TH PAURI OF JAPJI SAHIB

ਬਹੁਤਾ ਕਰਮੁ ਲਿਖਿਆ ਨਾ ਜਾਇ ॥
ਵਡਾ ਦਾਤਾ ਤਿਲੁ ਨ ਤਮਾਇ ॥
ਕੇਤੇ ਮੰਗਹਿ ਜੋਧ ਅਪਾਰ ॥
ਕੇਤਿਆ ਗਣਤ ਨਹੀ ਵੀਚਾਰੁ ॥
ਕੇਤੇ ਖਪਿ ਤੁਟਹਿ ਵੇਕਾਰ ॥
ਕੇਤੇ ਲੈ ਲੈ ਮੁਕਰੁ ਪਾਹਿ ॥
ਕੇਤੇ ਮੂਰਖ ਖਾਹੀ ਖਾਹਿ ॥
ਕੇਤਿਆ ਦੂਖ ਭੂਖ ਸਦ ਮਾਰ ॥
ਏਹਿ ਭਿ ਦਾਤਿ ਤੇਰੀ ਦਾਤਾਰ ॥
ਬੰਦਿ ਖਲਾਸੀ ਭਾਣੈ ਹੋਇ ॥
ਹੋਰੁ ਆਖਿ ਨ ਸਕੈ ਕੋਇ ॥
ਜੇ ਕੋ ਖਾਇਕੁ ਆਖਣਿ ਪਾਇ ॥
ਓਹੁ ਜਾਣੈ ਜੇਤੀਆ ਮੁਹਿ ਖਾਇ ॥
ਆਪੇ ਜਾਣੈ ਆਪੇ ਦੇਇ ॥
ਆਖਹਿ ਸਿ ਭਿ ਕੇਈ ਕੇਇ ॥
ਜਿਸ ਨੋ ਬਖਸੇ ਸਿਫਤਿ ਸਾਲਾਹ ॥
ਨਾਨਕ ਪਾਤਿਸਾਹੀ ਪਾਤਿਸਾਹੁ ॥੨੫॥

Bahutaa karam likhiaa na jaa-ay.
Vadaa dataa til na tamaay.
Kaytay mange jodh apaar.
Kaythaa ganat nahee veechaar.
Kaytay khap tuteh vikar.
Kaytay lai lai mukar paa-eh.
Kaytay moorakh khaahee khaa-eh.
Kaytiaa dookh bhookh sad maar.
Ay-eh bhe daat tayree daataar
Band khaalasee bhanai hoe.
Hor aakh na sakai koe.
Jay ko khaa-ik akhaan paae.
Oh jaanai jaytee-aa muh khaa-ay.
Aapay jaanay aapay day-eh.
Aakheh se bhe kay-ee kay-eh.
Jis no bakhsay siphat saalaah.
Naanak paatisaahee paatisaah.

From *Japji Sahib: The Song of the Soul* by Ek Ong Kaar Kaur Khalsa

There are so many karmic plays, it isn't possible to write them all.
The Great Giver withholds nothing—not even the tiniest sesame seed.
There are so many warriors begging to merge into Thee.
There are so many who are counting but never reflect on or see You.
So many are exhausted, having broken themselves on vice.
There are so many who take everything and then deny receiving.
So many foolish ones do nothing but stuff their face with food.
So many are continually beaten down by endless pain and hunger.
Even these are your Gifts to us, Great Giver.
Slavery. Freedom. Both come from You.
It isn't possible for anyone to say more than this.
If someone who likes the sound of his own voice tries to speak about this,
he'll be shamed in so many ways.
You, Yourself, know. You, Yourself, give.
Those who can speak of it this way are very few.
The ones You bless to meditatively and lovingly chant and sing Your wonders,
Nanak, these persons are the nobility of nobility.

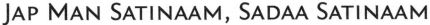

JAP MAN SATINAAM, SADAA SATINAAM

Siri Guru Granth Sahib ji, pages 669-670

This *shabad* brings prosperity and fulfills all desires.

ਧਨਾਸਰੀ ਮਹਲਾ ੪ ॥
ਇਛਾ ਪੂਰਕੁ ਸਰਬ ਸੁਖਦਾਤਾ ਹਰਿ ਜਾ ਕੈ ਵਸਿ ਹੈ ਕਾਮਧੇਨਾ ॥
ਸੋ ਐਸਾ ਹਰਿ ਧਿਆਈਐ ਮੇਰੇ ਜੀਅੜੇ ਤਾ ਸਰਬ ਸੁਖ ਪਾਵਹਿ ਮੇਰੇ ਮਨਾ ॥੧॥
ਜਪਿ ਮਨ ਸਤਿ ਨਾਮੁ ਸਦਾ ਸਤਿ ਨਾਮੁ ॥
ਹਲਤਿ ਪਲਤਿ ਮੁਖ ਊਜਲ ਹੋਈ ਹੈ ਨਿਤ ਧਿਆਈਐ ਹਰਿ ਪੁਰਖੁ ਨਿਰੰਜਨਾ ॥ ਰਹਾਉ ॥
ਜਹ ਹਰਿ ਸਿਮਰਨੁ ਭਇਆ ਤਹ ਉਪਾਧਿ ਗਤੁ ਕੀਨੀ ਵਡਭਾਗੀ ਹਰਿ ਜਪਨਾ ॥
ਜਨ ਨਾਨਕ ਕਉ ਗੁਰਿ ਇਹ ਮਤਿ ਦੀਨੀ ਜਪਿ ਹਰਿ ਭਵਜਲੁ ਤਰਨਾ ॥੨॥੬॥੧੨॥

Dhanaasree mehlaa 4.
Ichhaa poorak sarab sukh-daata har jaa kai vas hai kaamdhaynaa.
So aisaa har Dhi-aa-ee-ai mayray jee-arhay taa sarab sukh paavahi mayray manaa. ||1||
Jap man sat naam sadaa sat naam.
Halat palat mukh oojal ho-ee hai nit Dhi-aa-ee-ai har purakh niranjanaa. Rahaa-o.
Jah har simran bha-i-aa tah upaadh gat keenee vadbhaagee har japnaa.
Jan naanak ka-o gur ih mat deenee jap har bhavjal tarnaa. ||2||6||12||

Dhanaasaree, Fourth Mehl:
The Lord is the Fulfiller of desires, the Giver of total peace; the *Kaamadhaynaa*, the wish-fulfilling cow, is in His power.
So meditate on such a Lord, O my soul. Then, you shall obtain total peace, O my mind. ||1||
Chant, O my mind, the True Name, *Sat Nam*, the True Name.
In this world, and in the world beyond, your face shall be radiant, by meditating continually on the immaculate Lord God. ||Pause||
Wherever anyone remembers the Lord in meditation, disaster runs away from that place. By great good fortune, we meditate on the Lord.
The Guru has blessed servant Nanak with this understanding, that by meditating on the Lord, we cross over the terrifying world-ocean. ||2||6||12||

SOOKAY HARAY KEE-AY KHIN MAAHAY

Siri *Guru Granth Sahib ji*, page 191

This *shabad* brings prosperity and abundance.

ਗਉੜੀ ਮਹਲਾ ੫ ॥
ਸੁਕੇ ਹਰੇ ਕੀਏ ਖਿਨ ਮਾਹੇ ॥
ਅੰਮ੍ਰਿਤ ਦ੍ਰਿਸਟਿ ਸੰਚਿ ਜੀਵਾਏ ॥੧॥
ਕਾਟੇ ਕਸਟ ਪੂਰੇ ਗੁਰਦੇਵ ॥
ਸੇਵਕ ਕਉ ਦੀਨੀ ਅਪੁਨੀ ਸੇਵ ॥੧॥ ਰਹਾਉ ॥
ਮਿਟਿ ਗਈ ਚਿੰਤ ਪੁਨੀ ਮਨ ਆਸਾ ॥
ਕਰੀ ਦਇਆ ਸਤਿਗੁਰਿ ਗੁਣਤਾਸਾ ॥੨॥
ਦੁਖ ਨਾਠੇ ਸੁਖ ਆਇ ਸਮਾਏ ॥
ਢੀਲ ਨ ਪਰੀ ਜਾ ਗੁਰਿ ਫੁਰਮਾਏ ॥੩॥
ਇਛ ਪੁਨੀ ਪੂਰੇ ਗੁਰ ਮਿਲੇ ॥
ਨਾਨਕ ਤੇ ਜਨ ਸੁਫਲ ਫਲੇ ॥੪॥੫੮॥੧੨੭॥

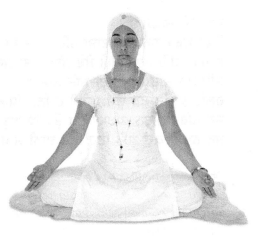

Ga-orhee mehlaa 5.
Sookay haray kee-ay khin maahay.
Amrit darisat sanch jeevaa-ay. ||1||
Kaatay kasat pooray gurdayv.
Sayvak ka-o deenee apunee sayv. ||1|| rahaa-o.
Mit ga-ee chint punee man aasaa.
Karee da-i-aa satgur guntaasaa. ||2||
Dukh naathay sukh aa-ay samaa-ay.
Dheel na paree jaa gur furmaa-ay. ||3||
Ichh punee pooray gur milay.
Naanak tay jan sufal falay. ||4||58||127||

Gauree, Fifth Mehl:
The dried branches are made green again in an instant.
His Ambrosial Glance irrigates and revives them. ||1||
The Perfect Divine Guru has removed my sorrow.
He blesses His servant with His service. ||1||Pause||
Anxiety is removed, and the desires of the mind are fulfilled,
When the True Guru, the Treasure of Excellence, shows His Kindness. ||2||
Pain is driven far away, and peace comes in its place;
There is no delay, when the Guru gives the Order. ||3||
Desires are fulfilled, when one meets the True Guru;
O Nanak, His humble servant is fruitful and prosperous. ||4||58||127||

Jee-a Jant Suprasan Bha-ay

Siri Guru Granth Sahib ji, page 716

This *shabad* brings relief from debts.

ਬਿਲਾਵਲੁ ਮਹਲਾ ੫ ॥
ਜੀਅ ਜੰਤ ਸੁਪ੍ਰਸੰਨ ਭਏ ਦੇਖਿ ਪ੍ਰਭ ਪਰਤਾਪ ॥
ਕਰਜੁ ਉਤਾਰਿਆ ਸਤਿਗੁਰੂ ਕਰਿ ਆਹਰੁ ਆਪ ॥੧॥
ਖਾਤ ਖਰਚਤ ਨਿਬਹਤ ਰਹੈ ਗੁਰ ਸਬਦੁ ਅਖੂਟ ॥
ਪੂਰਨ ਭਈ ਸਮਗਰੀ ਕਬਹੂ ਨਹੀ ਤੂਟ ॥੧॥ ਰਹਾਉ ॥
ਸਾਧਸੰਗਿ ਆਰਾਧਨਾ ਹਰਿ ਨਿਧਿ ਆਪਾਰ ॥
ਧਰਮ ਅਰਥ ਅਰੁ ਕਾਮ ਮੋਖ ਦੇਤੇ ਨਹੀ ਬਾਰ ॥੨॥
ਭਗਤ ਅਰਾਧਹਿ ਏਕ ਰੰਗਿ ਗੋਬਿੰਦ ਗੁਪਾਲ ॥
ਰਾਮ ਨਾਮ ਧਨੁ ਸੰਚਿਆ ਜਾ ਕਾ ਨਹੀ ਸੁਮਾਰੁ ॥੩॥
ਸਰਨਿ ਪਰੇ ਪ੍ਰਭ ਤੇਰੀਆ ਪ੍ਰਭ ਕੀ ਵਡਿਆਈ ॥
ਨਾਨਕ ਅੰਤੁ ਨ ਪਾਈਐ ਬੇਅੰਤ ਗੁਸਾਈ ॥੪॥੩੨॥੬੨॥

Bilaaval mehlaa 5.
Jee-a jant suparsan bha-ay daykh parabh partaap.
Karaj utaari-aa satguroo kar aahar aap. ||1||
Khaat kharchat nibhat rahai gur sabad akhoot.
Pooran bha-ee samagree kabhoo nahee toot. ||1|| rahaa-o.
Saadhsang aaraadhnaa har nidh aapaar.
Dharam arath ar kaam mokh daytay nahee baar. ||2||
Bhagat araadheh ayk rang gobind gupaal.
Raam naam Dhan sanchi-aa jaa kaa nahee sumaar. ||3||
Saran paray parabh tayree-aa parabh kee vadi-aa-ee.
Naanak ant na paa-ee-ai bay-ant gusaa-ee. ||4||32||62||

Bilaaval, Fifth Mehl:
All beings and creatures are totally pleased, gazing on God's glorious radiance.
The True Guru has paid off my debt; He Himself did it. ||1||
Eating and expending it, it is always available; the Word of the *Guru's Shabad* is inexhaustible.
Everything is perfectly arranged; it is never exhausted. ||1||Pause||
In the *saadh sangat*, the Company of the Holy, I worship and adore the Lord, the infinite treasure.
He does not hesitate to bless me with *dharmic* faith, wealth, sexual success and liberation. ||2||
The devotees worship and adore the Lord of the Universe with single-minded love.
They gather in the wealth of the Lord's Name, which cannot be estimated. ||3||
O God, I seek Your Sanctuary, the glorious greatness of God.
Nanak: Your end or limitation cannot be found, O Infinite World-Lord. ||4||32||62||

REALITY, PROSPERITY AND ECSTASY[54]

Meditation to the Aquarian musical affirmation *Reality, Prosperity and Ecstasy* created by Yogi Bhajan, recorded by Nirinjan Kaur

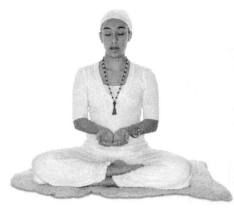

POSTURE: Sit in any meditative posture.

MUDRA: Hands are cupped together at the Navel Point.

EYES: Eyes are closed, focused at the tip of the nose.

CHANT: Sing to the musical affirmation *Reality, Prosperity and Ecstasy*.

COMMENTS: Prosperity never hurts. Contact it through the prosperity song; it shall happen. Prosperity means everything—richness in happiness, in our holiness and in our grace. This meditation is to experience richness in everything.

I know thou thee
Whaa-Hay Guroo Jee
Give my day
reality, prosperity
and ecstasy

54 This meditation and accompanying comments come from the private notes of Nirinjan Kaur, who served as Yogi Bhajan's Chief of Staff.

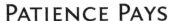

PATIENCE PAYS

Listen to the affirmation and guided meditation by Yogi Bhajan.

Patience pays. Wait. Let the hand of God work for you. The One who has created you—let Him create all the environments, circumstances, and facilities and faculties.

ਤੂ ਕਾਹੇ ਡੋਲਹਿ ਪ੍ਰਾਣੀਆ ਤੁਧੁ ਰਾਖੈਗਾ ਸਿਰਜਨਹਾਰੁ ॥
ਜਿਨਿ ਪੈਦਾਇਸਿ ਤੂ ਕੀਆ ਸੋਈ ਦੇਇ ਆਧਾਰੁ ॥੧॥

Too kaahay doleh paraanee-aa tudh raakhaigaa sirjanhaar.
Jin paidaa-is too kee-aa so-ee day-ay aadhaar. ||1||[55]

Oh individual why are you in a very doubtful state? The One who has made you will take care of you. The One who has created this Universe, all the planets, planetary faculties and facilities on Earth, He is the One who has created you. Wait. Have patience. Lean on Him. And all best things will come to you.

Dwell in God. Dwell in God. Dwell in God. Befriend your soul. Dwell in God and befriend your soul. Dwell in God and befriend your soul. Dwell in God and befriend your soul. All the faculties and facilities which are in your best interest shall be at your feet. You need million things? Million things will reach you. If you are stable, established, firm, patient. Remember, Creator watches over you. And creation is ready to serve you. If you just be you.

So please take away the ghost of your life and stop chasing round. Consolidate. Concentrate. Be you. And may all the peace, peaceful environments and prosperity approach you forever. Sat Nam.

---

55 Guru Arjan, Siri Guru Granth Sahib, page 724, line 6.

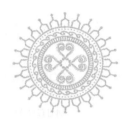

Part Five

Manifesting Success and Serving Others

FEEL YOUR ABUNDANCE
June 28, 2001

NOTE: There are no breaks between the exercises One, Two and Three.

PART ONE

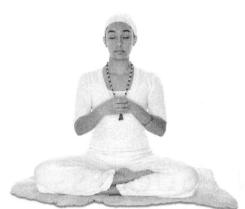

POSTURE: Sit in Easy Pose.

MUDRA: Make a fist of the left hand, with the thumb covering the fingers. Hold the fist 6 to 8 inches in front of the Heart Chakra and wrap the right hand around it. The palms are facing the body.

EYES: The eyes are closed.

BREATH: Long Deep Breathing.

TIME: 8 minutes.

PART TWO

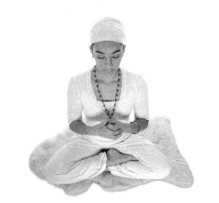

MUDRA: Now take the orange in both hands, and hold it as a symbol of prosperity.

EYE FOCUS: The eyes are focused at the tip of the nose. Be gracious.

TIME: 3 minutes.

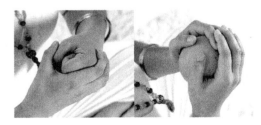

PART THREE

Peel the orange and eat it, chewing each bite very thoroughly. Take in the essence of prosperity.

COMMENTS: Feel yourself holding your abundance. The hand is your spirit. It is not a hand you are holding—it is Jupiter, Saturn, Sun and Mercury. The best thing in life is to know what you have. Sometimes we do not have the power to concentrate and we miss the opportunity. Elementary abundance is in your hands. Your hands will hold it, the breath of life, the breathing (prana) will be the longest possible, the maximum, and you will concentrate. That is all that is needed.

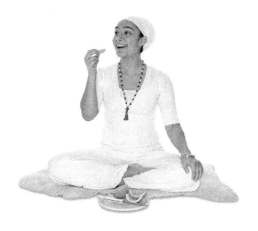

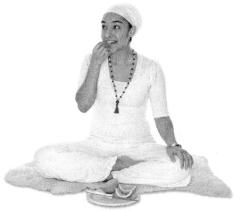

GURU NANAK'S TREASURE MEDITATION
February 11, 1978

"This meditation builds a deep sense of self-reliance. It allows you to separate your identity from your success."— Yogi Bhajan

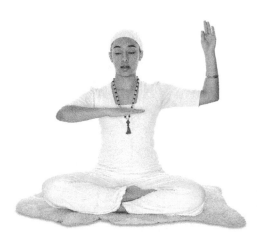

POSTURE: Sit in Easy Pose.

MUDRA: Raise the right arm in front of the Heart Center, bending the elbow so the forearm is parallel to the ground with the palm facing down. Raise the left arm out to the side of the body with the upper arm parallel to the ground, at shoulder level. Bend the elbow so the forearm is perpendicular to the ground with the fingers pointing up and palm facing forward as if you were taking an oath, the left hand in Gyan Mudra (index finger and thumb tip touching).

EYE FOCUS: The eyes are 1/10th open and focused the tip of the nose.

MANTRA: The entire mantra is repeated on a single breath. The tone is a relaxed monotone that varies in emphasis automatically as you proceed through the mantra.

HAR HAR HAR HAR HAREE HAREE.

Each *HAR* is one beat, and each *HAREE* is two beats.

TIME: Start with **11 minutes** and work up to **31 minutes**.

COMMENTS BY DR. GURUCHARAN SINGH KHALSA: This meditation builds a deep sense of self-reliance. It allows you to separate your identity from your success. It gives you potency, productivity and caliber. It makes you experience and believe in yourself. Then success comes to serve you, rather than you running after it. This meditation was taught by Guru Nanak then passed on by Baba Siri Chand and, later, by Guru Hargobind.

JUPITER KRIYA
TO BUILD BUSINESS INTUITION
February 4, 1990

"This kriya, called Jupiter Kriya, brings prosperity home. It is powerful enough to clear out the garbage in your subconscious mind. Your own electromagnetic psyche shall be tuned in with the Universal electromagnetic field." — Yogi Bhajan

PART ONE

POSTURE: Interlock the Jupiter fingers (index fingers), at the middle segment. The left index finger hooks down over the right. Bring the mudra to the Heart Center with the arms parallel to the ground. Holding the hands too low will cause depression. Keep the spine straight. Variation: you may also hold the mudra at the level of the Brow Point (between the eyebrows).

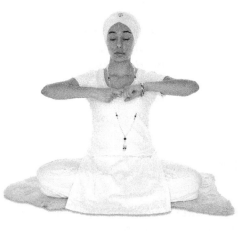

"If you hold the posture at the Heart Center, you will be an achiever. If you hold it at the Third Eye, you will have the strongest projection you can have." — Yogi Bhajan

EYE FOCUS: Fix your eyes at the tip of the nose. Totally relax your face.

BREATH: Make the lips round, as if you were sipping water. Then breathe deeply, inhaling through the mouth, exhaling through the nose. Breathe in like you are drinking in prosperity. Drink the *prana* (breath of life) through the mouth and exhale through the nose.

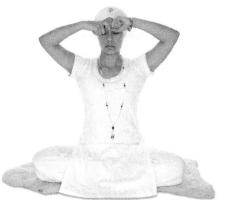

(continued on next page)

*Har Har Har Har
Gobinday
Har Har Har Har
Mukanday
Har Har Har Har
Udaaray
Har Har Har Har
Apaaray
Har Har Har Har
Hareeang
Har Har Har Har
Kareeang
Har Har Har Har
Nirnaamay
Har Har Har Har
Akaamay*

MANTRA: Listen deeply to the mantra *Har Har Har Har Gobinday* chanted by Nirinjan Kaur while you keep the breath going. The combined sound of the breath with the mantra guarantees prosperity. See translation on page 184.

COMMENTS: While you are meditating, ask for opportunities to flow into you.

TIME: If you are doing this meditation for **31 minutes**, continue Part One for **24 minutes**. If you are doing this meditation for **62 minutes**, continue Part One for **55 minutes**.

PART TWO

POSTURE: Keeping the Jupiter fingers interlocked, raise the arms and hold the mudra over the head above the Tenth Gate.

EYE FOCUS: Keep the eyes focused at the tip of the nose.

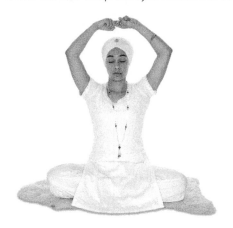

BREATH: Same as in Part One.

MANTRA: Same as Part One.

Continue for **5 minutes**, whether you are doing the meditation for 31 or 62 minutes.

This posture is done to establish brain strength. It will strengthen the grey matter. It creates a halo around your forehead—a sign of good luck.

PART THREE

POSTURE: Keeping the Jupiter fingers interlocked, lower the arms and hold the mudra at the Navel Center.

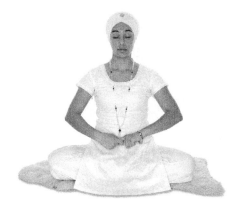

EYE FOCUS: Keep the eyes focused at the tip of the nose.

BREATH: Same as Part One.

MANTRA: Same as Part One.

Continue for **2 minutes**, whether you are doing the meditation for 31 or 62 minutes.

TO END: Shake the hands and your entire body very vigorously for **1 minute**. Every part of your body that you move will be your friend.

COMMENTS: In 3 minutes, the meditation will start breaking the blocks. Yawn or sneeze, but don't interfere with body language. You carry the tensions of years and years. Let them go. After approximately 11 minutes, the thought patterns in your head should start to change and your body should start to relax. With those tensions gone, you will start finding new horizons. About 15 minutes into the meditation, certain things that have been blocking you will start to tremble as the blocked energy is released. After approximately 22 minutes, you will start to face your mental blocks, which need your perfect attention. Keep the breath strong and full as the fight starts between you and your mind.

If you do this once a week for 62 minutes at a regular time, that's all you need. Within you there is a capacity to bring prosperity home. This kriya, called Jupiter Kriya, brings prosperity home. It is powerful enough to clear out the garbage in your subconscious mind. Your own electromagnetic psyche shall be tuned in with the Universal electromagnetic field. This will give you special energy and competence. There is hardly any possibility that you will have a problem. This meditation can be done for 31 minutes, out of kindness, but the requirement is to do it for 62 minutes.

Jupiter is the Lord of Knowledge. By holding the fingers in the Jupiter Lock, you will invoke the Jupiter guidance. By looking at the tip of your nose, you will control your mind to achieve it. By breathing a full breath—bringing in the *pranic* energy—you will bring the result home. Through the sound current, you will change the neurons of the brain to set a pattern of success. There is a subliminal, computerized permutation and combination in the sound of the mantra to assure prosperity.

RICHNESS WILL COME

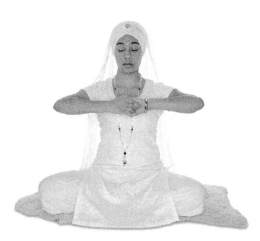

POSTURE: Sit in Easy Pose.

MUDRA: The hands are grasped tightly in front of the Heart Center in Bear Grip (the fingers of each hand are interlocked, left hand faces forward, right hand faces the chest). The forearms are parallel to the ground.

EYE FOCUS: Eyes are 1/10th open and focused the tip of the nose.

TIME: 11 to 31 minutes.

MANTRA:

Har Har Har Har Gobinday
Har Har Har Har Mukanday
Har Har Har Har Udaaray
Har Har Har Har Apaaray
Har Har Har Har Hareeang
Har Har Har Har Kareeang
Har Har Har Har Nirnamay
Har Har Har Har Akaamay

COMMENTS: This mantra (see translation on page 184) is to fix our mental relationship to prosperity and power. It will produce money; prosperity will come. Opportunities will come. Richness will come. It contains the eight facets of God that we all have to deal with.

Har is the *shakti* yog power mantra. *Har* is the original God. The repetitions of *Har* give power to all these facets, and provide the power to break down the past and barriers to our success.

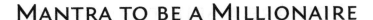

MANTRA TO BE A MILLIONAIRE

POSTURE: Sit in a meditative pose.

MUDRA: Not specified.

EYE FOCUS: Not specified.

MANTRA: Chant this brief *shabad* from the *Siri Guru Granth Sahib*, page 1193, line 7. *Basant Kee Vaar*, Fifth Mehl, Guru Arjan. See Yogi Bhajan's discussion of this mantra on page 86.

ਹਰਿ ਕਾ ਨਾਮੁ ਧਿਆਇ ਕੈ ਹੋਹੁ ਹਰਿਆ ਭਾਈ ॥
ਕਰਮਿ ਲਿਖੰਤੈ ਪਾਈਐ ਇਹ ਰੁਤਿ ਸੁਹਾਈ ॥

Har kaa naam

Dhi-aa-ay kai hohu hari-aa bhaa-ee.

Karam likhantai paa-ee-ai ih rut suhaa-ee.

TRANSLATION:
Contemplating God's Name,
Flower, thou, my brother.
In accordance with the write of destiny
Thou are blessed with this beauteous
season.

TIME: Chant **11 times** a day.

YOU ARE A SPIRITUAL BEING WITH UNLIMITED POTENTIAL

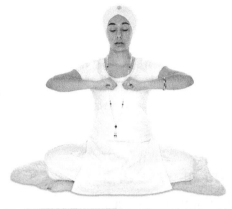

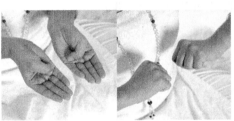

POSTURE: Sit in Easy Pose.

MUDRA: Bring the thumbs to touch the mound of the Mercury finger (pinkie) and fold the fingers over the thumb to make tight fists. Bring the forearms parallel to the floor at the Heart Center. Knuckles face each other with a one-inch gap between the hands.

EYE FOCUS: Focus the eyes on the tip of the nose.

MANTRA: Chant *HAR* **4 times out loud, 4 times in a whisper** continuously. Make sure the tongue flicks up to the upper palate.

TIME: 11-21 minutes.

COMMENTS BY DR. GURUCHANDER SINGH KHALSA: This meditation contains the ego and allows you to focus on your true identity as a spiritual being with unlimited potential and self-worth. When we put the thumb (ego) at the mound of the Mercury finger, we transform our ego identity through the influence of Mercury, Sun, Saturn and Jupiter. This transformation includes mastering expansion (Jupiter), wisdom and patience (Saturn), endurance (Sun) and communication (Mercury) towards our spiritual identity. We use the mantra *HAR* to bring new opportunities into our life. By creating mastery at the Heart Center, we can transform our passion and heart energy into personal and financial success within our spiritual life. Remember—doing meditations creates the opportunity to change our attitudes towards our world. When you do this meditation for at least 120 days, your subconscious can shift into a larger, more expansive attitude about being prosperous (pro-spirit).

TOUCH OTHERS
December 20, 1997

POSTURE: Sit in Easy Pose.

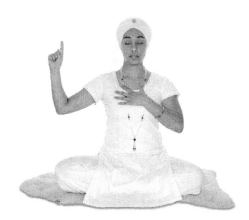

MUDRA: Spread the fingers of the left hand as far apart as possible and place the hand on the Heart Center with the thumb pointing up. Make the right hand into a fist with the index finger extended. Place the right arm by the side with the elbow down and the index finger pointing up. Position the arm so that the tip of the right index finger is level with the tip of the eye, palm facing forward.

EYES: Eyes are closed.

BREATH: Long Deep Breathing.

MANTRA: After relaxing into the breath, begin chanting the Kundalini Shakti mantra.

AAD SACH, JUGAAD SACH, HAI BHEE SACH, NAANAK HOSEE BHEE SACH

Pull the navel powerfully each time you chant *"sach"* so that the belly button connects with the spine. Continue for at least **8 minutes**.

In class, Yogi Bhajan said that different people might need to practice this meditation for different durations.

> **TRANSLATION:**
> True in the beginning,
> True throughout the Ages
> True at this moment,
> Nanak says this Truth
> shall ever be.

TO END: Inhale deeply. Exhale and relax.

COMMENTS: We touch each other with the eyes. We touch each other with the ears. We touch each other with songs and words. We touch physically. We touch to kill. We touch to give birth. If you look at the whole spectrum of life, it's nothing but touch. If you want to know the Master's Touch, then you should live these words of Nanak.

This is called the combination of polarities: your breath has a length of thirty-six inches. When you press the navel to create the word sound *"sach,"* after a long practice or a short practice—depending on your habit—you become intuitive. Provided all five fingers on the left hand are open and the right hand index finger is up.

MEDITATION FOR INTERDEPENDENCE
November 6, 1990

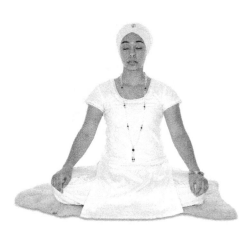

POSTURE: Sit in Easy Pose, hands in any relaxed position, make a strong clucking sound with your tongue striking and releasing against the upper palate. The tongue presses the upper palate and breaks from it with a force. It pulls forcefully on the upper palate at the rate of approximately 2 clucks per second.

TIME: NOT MORE THAN **3 minutes.**

COMMENTS: The person most slave-like is the one who is trying to prove he is independent—because life is totally interdependent.

Nobody can afford the thought to be independent because even our life is dependent on our breath. Dependency starts on that which this body lives. How independent can you be? Your life depends upon the central ear. There are three bones. One hammer bone strikes the other bone. If that bone stops hammering, you're done. Your whole world of listening depends on your two ears. Your whole universe depends on your two eyes, whether you see or not. If your two nostrils stop breathing, you are dead. Within us still we say, "I want to be independent. I want to prove it to everybody." Prove what and to whom? There is a certain reality in us, a certain depth in us, a certain self in us. If we enlarge that then we can overcome.

The idea of life is prosperity. Prosperity does not mean that you have a lot of money and you sit on it. Beauty is not just that you look young and beautiful and charming and sensual and sexual. Beauty is many things: beauty in manners, beauty in behavior, beauty in personality, and beauty in making the deals and dealing with people. Every aspect that is wonderful and beyond wonderful is beautiful. Every human that acts to answer the call of duty in a perfectly direct or indirect manner is the most beautiful human in relationship to that act. That is how life is and that is how we have to live life.

Stimulate your hypothalamus by doing this exercise but please don't do it more than three minutes. More than three minutes and it's no longer an exercise, it becomes an addiction. I'd like to go on record and warn you that you are entitled to do it for three minutes only.

PROSPERITY MANDALA

By meditating on the Prosperity Mandala, you will understand the transient nature of life, and its cycles. Infinite blessings will flow to you. Place the Prosperity Mandala in an important location in your home and chant the prosperity mantra (translation available on page 184):

Har Har Har Har
Gobinday
Har Har Har Har
Mukanday
Har Har Har Har
Udaaray
Har Har Har Har
Apaaray
Har Har Har Har
Hareeang
Har Har Har Har
Kareeang
Har Har Har Har
Nirnaamay
Har Har Har Har
Akaamay

To see and order a copy of the Prosperity Mandala, visit www.sikhdharma.org.

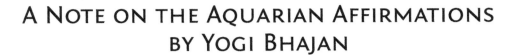

A NOTE ON THE AQUARIAN AFFIRMATIONS BY YOGI BHAJAN

A Note on Aquarian Musical Affirmations by Yogi Bhajan, recorded by Nirinjan Kaur

Yogi Bhajan personally directed these recordings for their specific meditative effects on the subconscious and the nervous system.

Over the years he said many things about them. Here are some of his comments about their impact and effect.

"The recordings are based on the *Adi Naad* sound system, the *Adi* word hypnotic sound affirmation. These hypnotic affirmations uplift the inner soul. They open the chakras and stimulate the balance of the five *tattvas*.

"By opening up the seven chakras, we can access our inner force which is gifted with intuition. Nirinjan Kaur has a God-given, precious gift to create this hypnotic *naad*.

"When you listen to these recordings, a vibration is created in the drum of your ear. The message stimulates the subconscious mind, which releases its subconscious blocks and stimulates conscious activity. Then the human has a victory of unconscious withdrawals. It is the most wonderful self-realization system.

"These hypnotic affirmations stimulate the meridians of the upper palate through the permutation and combination of the sound. If the individual sings along while practicing or playing these recordings, they further stimulate the hypothalamus. The neurons in the brain are readjusted for the beautiful, bountiful, blissful success of the individual. It is a God-given gift for you and for your prosperity. The system works. It shall work for you.

"The affirmations are designed to burn negative karma and stimulate positive inspiration. Many people have tried it. It has worked miracles. Miracles are unexplainable wonderful happenings. They are not gimmicks or soul talk. They are a reality that can be proven by the practicing practitioner.

"It is the word that elevates the human. The word solves and dissolves problems, gives peace of mind, happiness, fulfillment of destiny and prosperity. When you know the right permutation and combination of words, you can open up every lock and cross every hurdle of life. You can have a happy, prosperous life and gain a beautiful, bountiful and blissful status.

"These are very special recordings for ordinary people to become special. Honestly use them in your life for 120 days and you will feel happy and prosperous.

In the case of specific difficulties, all you have to do is to take the recording and have it on continuous play. Put it on at night and sleep. It is a very effective way to remove the blocks from the subconscious."

A NOTE ON THE AQUARIAN AFFIRMATIONS BY YOGI BHAJAN

APPENDIX A

Effects of Shabads from the Siri Guru Granth Sahib

In the meditation section of this book, there are *shabad*s and lines from *shabad*s that come from the *Siri Guru Granth Sahib*. As a master of Kundalini Yoga, Yogi Bhajan would sense how the sound current of a particular *shabad* could remove specific obstacles or bring about a particular result. His description of the effect of a *shabad* is included with the *shabad*, itself.

These descriptions are not part of the Yogi Bhajan Library of Teachings; nor do they necessarily coincide with the historical understanding of the *Siri Guru Granth Sahib* found in the mainstream Sikh community. However, based on Yogi Bhajan's descriptions, many people over the years have experienced the benefits of these *shabad*s through their own meditation. We are grateful to make this information—which he shared during his lifetime—available to you.

For more information on *Sikh Dharma, Shabad Guru* and the *Siri Guru Granth Sahib*, visit www.sikhdharma.org.

APPENDIX B

Lecture Dates

The chapters in this book draw from the following lectures given by Kundalini Yoga master Yogi Bhajan, also known as the Siri Singh Sahib of *Sikh Dharma*.

Chapter 1: December 26, 1997
Chapter 2: April 24, 1991
Chapter 3: October 3, 1996
Chapter 4: November 19, 2000 and November 10, 2001
Chapter 5: April 30, 2001
Chapter 6: October 16, 1993
Chapter 7: July 25, 1989
Chapter 8: April 15, 1988
Chapter 9: March 5, 1995 and September 4. 2001
Chapter 10: September 10, 1995 and January 17, 2000
Chapter 11: April 14, 1992
Chapter 12: June 28, 2001
Chapter 13: April 19, 1989
Chapter 14: October 22, 1994
Chapter 15: December 20, 1997 and June 21, 2001

To learn more about the Yogi Bhajan Library of Teachings,
visit www.kundaliniresearchinstitute.org.

INDEX

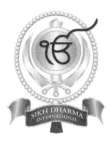

About Sikh Dharma International

The Sikh religion began in India more than 530 years ago. Since then Sikhs from the Punjab, who make up less than 2 percent of India's population, have migrated throughout Europe, the Americas, and Asia, numbering about 28 million around the world. In the early 1970s, Yogi Bhajan, who would later be known as Siri Singh Sahib Bhai Sahib Harbhajan Singh Khalsa Yogiji, began to teach in the United States. Through his inspiration, insight and example many Westerners began adopting the Sikh way of life, attracted by the spiritual practices of Sikh Dharma and its egalitarian teachings that respect all religions and all peoples.

One aspect of our mission is to preserve, organize and continue to share the teachings of the Sikh Gurus as described by the late Siri Singh Sahib in his unique style. His way of teaching about the Sikh path has, for the first time in history, made the Sikh tradition accessible to people from every background, language, and culture of the world.

In addition to this primary mission, Sikh Dharma International maintains the principles of Sikh Dharma as it's understood around the world: We do not convert people; but we do serve. Sikh populations everywhere participate enthusiastically in outreach activities and contribute to their surrounding communities. The Sikh teachings encourage people to live their lives in service to others from a place of abundance, peace, and prosperity. Sikhs not only serve humanity and but also build interfaith dialogue and cooperation among all peoples.

For more than 40 years Sikh Dharma International (SDI) has been a recognized non-profit 501c(3) religious organization in the United States.

To learn more about Sikh Dharma International, visit www.sikhdharma.org.

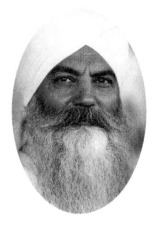

About Yogi Bhajan

In the late 1960s, the West was going through a revolution of consciousness. The young people of the time had a longing to touch Divinity. An Indian Kundalini Yoga Master who would come to be known as "Yogi Bhajan," answered their call and traveled to the West in 1968. For the first time in recorded history, he openly taught Kundalini Yoga, a very old and sacred science for awakening God-consciousness within the individual. He often said that he had come to the West "to create teachers, not to gain students."

Yogi Bhajan was not only a Master of Kundalini Yoga, but he was also a Sikh. As thousands of people flocked to study yoga with him, a smaller group of his students became fascinated by the Sikh tradition. One by one, through his inspiration and example, they began to adopt the Sikh way of life, Sikh Dharma.

Through his personal efforts, Sikh Dharma was officially recognized as a religion in the United States in 1971. That same year, in recognition of his extraordinary impact of spreading the universal message of Sikh Dharma, he was given the title Siri Singh Sahib, Chief Religious and Administrative Authority for the Western Hemisphere and given the responsibility to create a Sikh Ministry in the West. He was later honored with the title, Bhai Sahib, in 1974.

Founded in compassion, and a commitment to sharing teachings that would help free people from their pain and confusion, Yogi Bhajan carried out his mission for nearly 40 years. Under his spiritual guidance, ashrams, yoga centers, Gurdwaras and communities sprang up all over the world. He was also a pioneer in the interfaith movement and a friend and mentor to public leaders everywhere.

From 1968 until his death on October 6, 2004, Yogi Bhajan traveled, taught, and inspired millions around the world. His work had such far-reaching impact that after his death, a special bipartisan Joint Resolution was issued by the United States Congress honoring his life and work. He taught that God lives in everyone and everything. And that to experience the Divine is the privileged, right and ultimate aim of every human life.

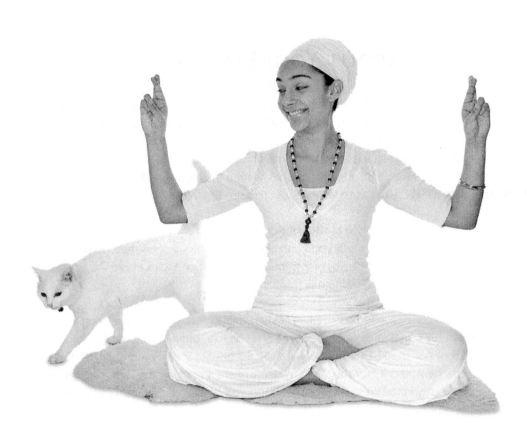

CPSIA information can be obtained at www.ICGtesting.com
Printed in the USA
LVOW03s0958070514

384766LV00004B/8/P